'HOW TO'

BOOK OF

FITNESS

& EXERCISE

DR. VAUGHAN THOMAS

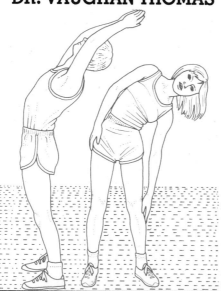

BLANDFORD PRESS
POOLE, DORSET

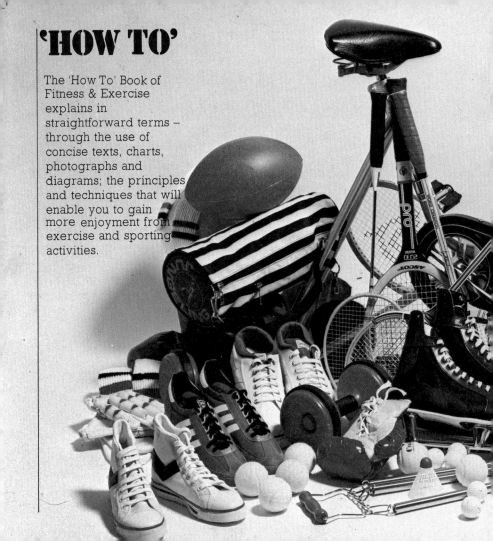

'HOW TO'

The 'How To' Book of Fitness & Exercise explains in straightforward terms – through the use of concise texts, charts, photographs and diagrams; the principles and techniques that will enable you to gain more enjoyment from exercise and sporting activities.

Contents

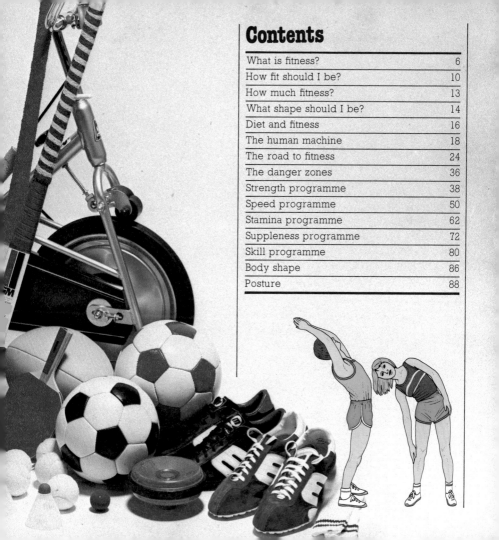

The 'How To' Book of Fitness and
Exercise was conceived, edited and
designed by Simon Jennings and Company Limited,
42 Maiden Lane, London WC2, England

General Editor: Michael Bowers

Art Direction: Simon Jennings

Text: Dr Vaughan Thomas

Illustrations: Coral Mula

Special Photography: John Couzins

Design and Research Assistant: Caroline Peacocke

First published in the United Kingdom 1981
Copyright © 1981 Blandford Press Limited
Link House, West Street, Poole,
Dorset BH15 1LL, England

Text and Illustrations Copyright
© 1981 Simon Jennings and Company Limited

ISBN 0 7137 1047 0
Printed in Singapore

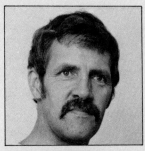

THE AUTHOR

Dr Vaughan Thomas is
the head of the
Department of Sport and
Recreation Studies at
Liverpool Polytechnic
and the author of seven
books on sport, science
and positive health. He
has also published over
60 research papers in
this field. His own
sporting career has been
distinguished, achieving
international standard at
athletics, basket ball and
cycling. At the age of 45,
he continues to be a
successful sportsman at a
high level of competition.
Dr Thomas is also an
accomplished musician.

Introduction

Living in industrialised 'developed' societies exposes man to two conflicting forces which affect his physical well being. On the one hand, the enormous and ever accelerating rate of medical research has virtually created an environment in which no one need die of infectious disease. Just a short time ago in the history of man, infection was the biggest natural killer by far. Nowadays, anyone living in a developed society has access to a system of preventative medicine which can just about assure him of reaching his full life span of three score years and ten.

On the other hand, the relative affluence of the developed society, and the decreasing necessity to engage in really hard physical work, means that man is exposed to other killers which were almost unknown to our ancestors. These two modern plagues are physical idleness and food fetishism. Because technological man gets insufficient exercise, his heart becomes progressively weak until one day it is faced with a task beyond its capacity – and just stops. Secondly, since consuming food, drink and drugs is pleasant, affluent man does more of it than is strictly necessary. This causes his body to become too big and inefficient for his out of condition engine to handle.

Throughout history the average man has been stronger and fitter than the average man of today. The English archers of Agincourt used bows which even the modern competitive archer could not pull! Historical man, honed to a fine pitch by his physical existence, was quite capable of living a full life span. The high death rate from infectious disease meant that the overall average life span was greatly diminished, but if he escaped that early 'plague' the chances of reaching a ripe old age were, if anything, greater than those of modern man.

Even though the medical profession has *added years to our life*, it is up to us to *add life to our years*. Society has given us an opportunity to enjoy a long life; we must surely make it a good one. In fact, a life which is FIT to live. A part of that fitness for life concerns our physical selves. This is 'Physical Fitness', and this book aims to show you how to achieve it. Enjoyably, safely, and profitably; but above all – effectively and efficiently, since fitness should not be an end in itself, but a key which opens many doors to happiness and fulfilment.

What is fitness?

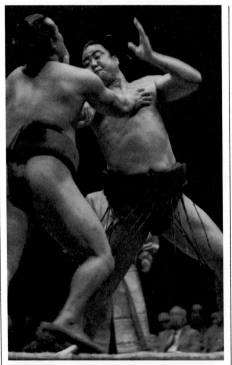

Though it is a hackneyed thing to say, there are as many meanings to fitness as there are individuals. *Fitness* as a word or a concept is rather like *goodness* or *beauty*. What one person perceives as being good or beautiful, another may consider bad or ugly. The kind of fitness admired by the Japanese sumo wrestler is a gross travesty of fitness to a long distance runner. There are no absolute standards of fitness, no golden yardsticks against which each individual can judge himself.

If we start with the word 'fit', we find that it refers to the possession of some desirable qualities. I am 'fit' to be your friend if I possess those qualities which you admire; a square peg is not 'fit' for a round hole; the lyrics of a song 'fit' the music.

We can only define fitness if we specify which physical qualities are desirable. And these qualities are absolutely specific to each individual and his life style. It would be a huge confidence trick for this book to lay out a fitness charter for every reader. What it can do is to make clear and interesting the basic principles, and show the reader how to work out his own physical destiny in the way which fits him.

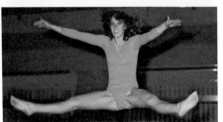

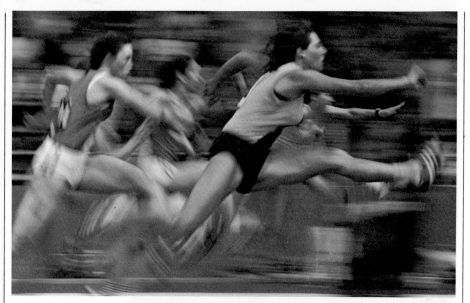

The Sumo wrestler *top left* has fitness, though his bulk may seem to contradict that. The other end of the scale is represented by the gymnast who requires total suppleness and therefore has no bulk at all. The hurdlers, *above*, combine power with suppleness and are generally more muscular than gymnasts. Swimmers, *right*, typify a combination of strength and stamina.

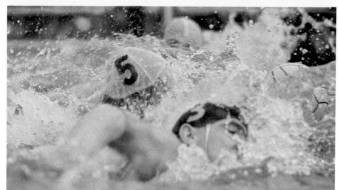

General fitness

When people think of physical fitness, in most cases it is *general fitness* which they understand. This is seen as a kind of all-embracing state of body, suitable for everyone, and capable of being turned to any task. A panacea of positive health, in fact.

The best way to look at general fitness is to discover what physical needs are general amongst nearly all normal people. By gradually stripping away those needs which are specific to certain special classes of people, we are left with those which we all need to be concerned about.

The first, and most important, thing is that we want to be alive and capable of functioning physically. This involves maintaining a constant and sufficient supply of *fuel* and *oxygen* to all parts of the body. The system which accomplis-

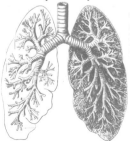

The Lungs
Oxygen is one of the body's major needs. Fitness demands that the lungs, which supply the body with oxygen, function to their maximum efficiency. Training will improve their capacity.

hes this comprises the heart, lungs and blood vessels.

The second element of general fitness is concerned with our ability to do *work*, in the sense which an engineer would understand. That is, to be able to exert forces on ourselves or on external objects, causing them to move or to remain steady against some opposing force. This element is concerned with the muscles of the body. As far as general fitness goes, muscles should be able to cope with the general activities of life – walking, occasionally running, climbing stairs, lifting heavy weights, unscrewing tightly fastened objects, pushing against resistances, maintaining certain postures for long periods of time, and so on.

The third aspect of general fitness defines our body's capacity to assume various shapes. If our muscles and joints are stiff and unyielding we have difficulty in reaching some extreme positions, like touching the floor with the hands (when gardening for example), or washing one's back, or doing modern dances. Even sexual performance can be less enjoyable if participants lack physical suppleness.

Fourthly, general fitness includes an

ability to perform physical tasks with *skill* and efficiency. Modern living is full of required physical tasks. Manipulative skills like handwriting, using cutlery, shaving or making up, can be performed more skilfully by proper practice. Driving vehicles constitutes a most complex skill. Even reading a book like this is a physical skill which is badly performed by many people. Also repetitive skills, like walking or peeling potatoes, can be performed very inefficiently, wasting much energy which leads to early fatigue.

Most people recognise the fifth element of general fitness – the ability to move quickly. In reality, this element is composed of two distinct parts. The first can be called *Reaction* – the ability to respond quickly to any particular situation or stimulus. Examples of this in general living are braking your vehicle in emergency, blinking to avoid an attacking fly, catching baby when he falls. The second element of speed is *Velocity* – the ability to move over a distance in a short space of time. Running for a bus, catching a lift, are good examples of this.

The last element of general fitness is the most difficult to understand. If the body is a physical machine (which it is) then something is needed to make it work – to motivate it, in fact. When the physical going gets tough; when every fibre says 'this is impossible – stop – enough'; when pain, boredom, fear and a hundred other emotions born of physical stress are pleading with you to slow down and rest; this is when the *spirit* of the generally fit person refuses to give in, and shifts the individual into a new domain of performance. With a highly developed spirit barriers recede, obstacles melt, and Man becomes Superman.

These are days of sensation seeking, through drugs, media, pornography, and so on. Yet how few people in our sedentary and pampered society experience one of the greatest sensations of all. Being really fit is like being permanently 'high' but without the ill effects of most of the popular sensations. And like a drug trip, a sexual orgasm, a religious conversion, a political coup engineered, a big business deal clinched – until you have experienced it you can have little idea of what the feeling is like.

This book will show you how to get that feeling, and keep it for life!

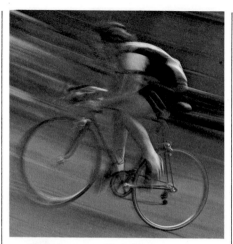

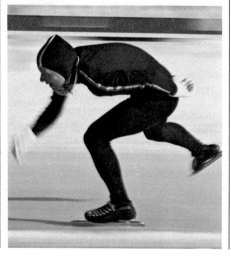

How fit should I be?

That question must have been posed millions of times to fitness advisers of all kinds, qualified or ·unqualified. And what so few of these self-styled experts realise is that the response must be another question.... 'What do you want to do?' Even if the answer is a simple 'I want to be generally fit for my sedentary life style', there are still questions to be asked. 'Do you live in a high rise flat, or a house with a garden?' 'What age, body build and which sex are you?' 'Do you own a car?' 'Do you live in town or country?' 'Do you work in an office or factory?' 'Do you have any hereditary physical defects?' The list is never ending. How long is a ray of light?

But of course the individual also has his own specific fitness needs, over and above his general fitness. These may be concerned with his work and his leisure, and it is interesting that most people perform harder physical work in their leisure time than they do in their employment. The elements described under *General Fitness* apply equally well to specific fitness. We can remind ourselves of them, noting that they begin with S: Stamina, Strength, Suppleness, Skill, Speed, Spirit; the Six S's.

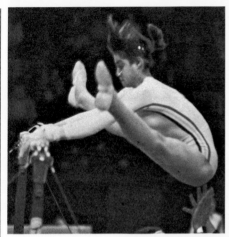

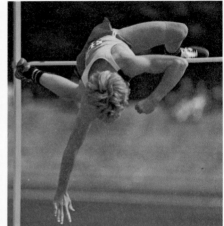

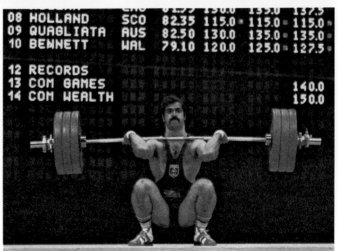

A gymnast, *above left*, must combine extreme suppleness with skill. High jumpers are certainly supple but their event does not require the range of techniques used in gymnastics. Weightlifting, *right*, requires great strength, but of a short 'explosive' nature. These big men, and others such as shot putters, often possess considerable speed. But it is a very different speed to that of the skater, *bottom left*. Racing cyclists, *top left*, must possess both speed and stamina.

08	HOLLAND	ENG	81.99	130.0	135.0	137.5
09	QUAGLIATA	SCO	82.35	115.0	115.0	115.0
10	BENNETT	AUS	82.50	130.0	135.0	135.0
		WAL	79.10	120.0	125.0	127.5
12	RECORDS					
13	COM GAMES					140.0
14	COM WEALTH					150.0

Fit for what?

Not many of us know ourselves very well. We may occasionally embark on an orgy of introspection of our own motives, or emotions, or personality. But as far as our physical life is concerned, we are surprisingly ignorant. It is difficult to specify what we are going to be fit for. So, a little analysis is called for, and it will be helpful to be well organised in that analysis. If we design a chart, with the six S's along one side, and our usual physical activities listed down the other, we can form what is called a matrix of cells. In each cell we can make at least one arbitrary guess of how much activity we do – or would like to do. As long as the really significant physical activities in one's life are included, then a reasonable answer to the question 'how much?' can be estimated. At least in relative terms, the importance of strength against speed can be gauged, and also the relative importance of work activities against leisure.

THE SIX S'S

Check your routine
The chart shows how certain selected activities score against the six S's. The value, or requirement, under each heading is expressed on a scale of 1–10. For example, a shop assistant who performed all the listed activities in one day would score well for stamina and spirit, moderately well for skill, but no better than average for strength.

Activity	DAILY ROUTINE Working 8 hours	Sleeping 8 hours	Cycling to work 1 hour	Playing squash 1 hour	Visiting pub 1 hour	Watching TV 1·5 hours	D.I.Y. 1 hour	Reading 1 hour	Miscellaneous 1·5 hours	Average Daily value
STAMINA	7	0	7	10	2	4	6	2	3	10
STRENGTH	2	0	6	7	1	3	7	1	3	5
SUPPLENESS	2	0	3	7	1	2	5	1	3	4·5
SKILL	3	0	6	10	1	5	9	1	3	7
SPEED	2	0	7	10	0	1	5	0	3	5
SPIRIT	5	0	7	10	1	1	7	1	3	8

How much fitness?

Eventually, for almost all individuals, the question has to be answered indirectly. Since fitness is achieved only by expenditure of time and energy, the only real limits to how much fitness a person is capable of achieving are set by the amount of time and energy he can allocate. This allocation needs to be spent wisely and effectively.

More is not always better

It would be very difficult to argue against the concept that a fitter heart and lungs, even greater skill, and stronger spirit would always be desirable in terms of general fitness. But in the case of speed and strength, the general limit would be reached at a relatively low level. Sprinting for buses does not figure so prominently in the life of Mr. Average that ever increasing sprinting speeds are going to be terribly useful, and ever greater strength is normally accompanied by ever bigger muscles which might be considered an unsightly or bulky nuisance by all except the body builder! In the case of suppleness, the point is even more critical. Most joints of the body are protected by strong fibrous 'cords' called ligaments, which prevent a joint from flexing so far that it becomes unstable. Extreme suppleness is achieved by stretching these ligaments, making the joints potentially unstable.

Specificity – What sort of training?

The fitness matrix for each person not only determines how much fitness but also, since fitness is acquired by training, how much' training. Even more important, it also determines what form the training will take. For utmost effectiveness, training should be specific. The specificity applies in two ways.

Firstly, training for specific activities should involve a large component of actually doing the activity. Training for running must involve running, training for strength must involve heavy exercises, training for swimming must involve getting wet. Though many professional soccer players play golf as part of their training, it is of doubtful value apart from psychological relaxation.

Secondly, general training of (say) the heart must also produce the specific desired effects on the heart. In this case, it does not matter at all to the heart whether the activity is running, swimming, or playing squash. What matters is the duration, intensity and frequency of the exercise.

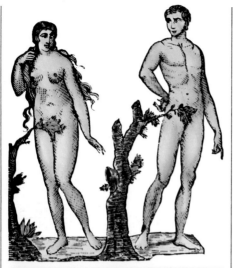

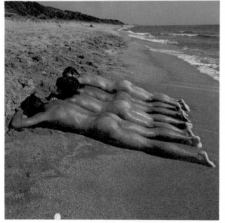

What shape should I be?

We have two shapes. The one given us by our parents at birth, and the one developed from that by our lifestyle, i.e. our *natural* and our *developed shapes*. We can always change our developed shape, by exercise and diet, but never our natural shape, which is the shape we 'should be'. There are three basic patterns for humans: linear, wedge and round. *(see page 86)*

These patterns are caused by our bone structure, our tendency for big muscles, and our efficiency at processing food. The latter two are affected by our life style, which provides us with the opportunity of developing the shape we want, within limits set by our inherited pattern. Anyone can be a Bodybuilder.

In children the picture is more complicated because rates at which the various parts of their pattern develop are different. And, while we can speak of typical shapes at certain ages, these are merely averages from a wide spread range. Quite normal children can vary by several years from the typical growth rate without any harm whatsoever. By the time they have finished growing they will have returned to somewhere near the average.

Our basic natural shape, *right*, is unalterable, but it can and will be developed by our life-style. Our shape may then look very different, *below*. If we choose to be fit we will have some choice in the way that our bodies develop, but we will not be able to change our natural shape. In other words, a wedge shaped person will always be wedge shaped, but he or she can develop any part of the body at will. We may want to look good in public, *far left*; the motive may be vanity, but the fitness is beneficial.

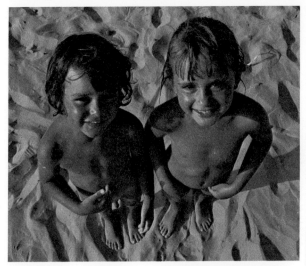

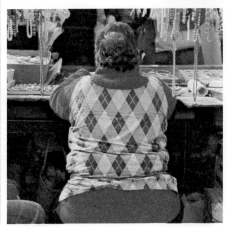

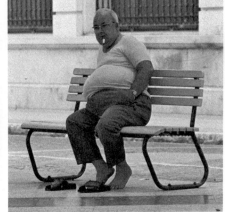

15

Diet and fitness

The things we consume (food, drink, drugs, pollution) have certain effects on us:

1. They provide fuel for the human machine; 2. They build and replace body tissues; 3. They fight infection and keep us healthy; 4. They give us pleasure and satisfaction; Or 5. They poison us.

Quite clearly, we need an amount of fuel which exactly equals the amount of energy we expend; we need enough to build the shape we want and to keep it there by replacing worn parts; we need a very small amount to keep us healthy; and as little of that which poisons us as possible. That total intake is what we need. Any more, and we get FAT – any less, and we get THIN.

It is important to realise that hardly anyone has the rare medical condition which prevents him from obeying this rule of diet. But we do vary in our efficiency as food processing machines. Those who are very efficient can get more benefit from the food they eat – so they need less food. Those who are efficient are the lucky ones, but if they eat the same as everyone else, they become fat. If they are sensible they eat less and better, or less and cheaper.

Diet and Exercise
Many people who embark on a programme of exercise with the intention of losing weight are disappointed with the results. Unfortunately, the greater food processing efficiency which comes with greater fitness is capable of cancelling out the weight loss benefits of exercise. Some even gain weight during the early days of exercising. Later on, if the fitness programme is progressive, there may be some loss of weight. But the only sure route to slimness is to eat less.

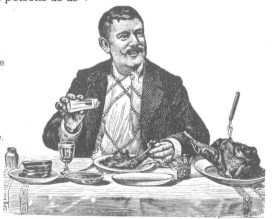

Food for sport

Though the performances of a sportsman may be exceptional, they are still natural. The actual food requirements of a sportsman are different from those of a sedentary person only in terms of *quantity* and *balance*. They are no different from, for example, an old fashioned lumberjack, a rickshaw puller, or any other really physically demanding occupation. On the other hand, food does have a psychological value, and if a sportsman can be made to believe that some magic diet can create superhuman abilities in him – then they will!

Virtually everything you eat and drink can provide you with energy. Purely in terms of quantity, the sportsman should eat food which he enjoys, and which does not lie heavily on his stomach, while working hard. The actual amount will depend on his total energy needs, divided into his 'vegetative' needs (necessary just to keep him alive); his 'human' needs, for all his non sporting activities; and his 'sporting' needs – training and competition. And, just as with every human being, the weighing machine will tell him whether he is consuming the right amount.

Your Energy needs
You will see from the chart that sportsmen, on the whole, have higher energy requirements than non sportsmen. This is only true of people undergoing heavy and demanding training schedules. Sport taken casually, with the minimum of preparation, drastically reduces the requirement.

NON SPORTSMEN	Food Requirements Kcals (calories)
Pensioners	2,300
Sedentary workers	2,500
Students	2,900
Building workers	3,000
Farmers	3,500
Miners	3,600
SPORTSMEN	**Food Requirements Kcals (calories)**
Sprinters	4,600
Games players	5,600
Long distance sports	6,000
Heavy power sports	7,000

The human machine

Packed into our bodies is a machine more complicated than a spacecraft, with an energy system more sophisticated than a nuclear power station, and an information network which would need a computer the size of a factory to reproduce. All of it motivated by a spirit which is unique and intangible. Let's take a look at the machine, the power station and the computer!

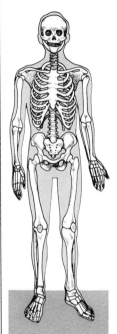

▲
Bone structure

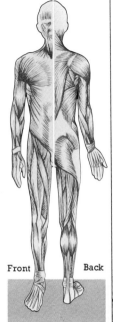

Front   Back

▲
Skeletal muscles

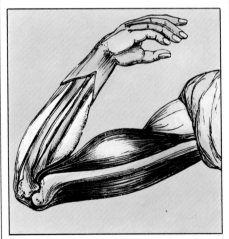

Muscular movement
The only actions that muscles perform is to pull against the bones to which they are attached.

The Machine
The bones form the framework of the body. Muscles, which transmit motive power, are attached to the bones. When stimulated by nerves, the 'elastic' fibres of the muscles contract, pulling and moving the bones to which they are attached. The mucles can only act in this way, so we have 215 pairs of them to cope with all the movements we have to make.

18

POWER STATION   COMPUTER

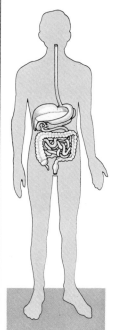

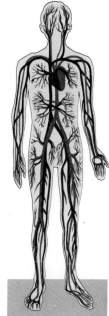

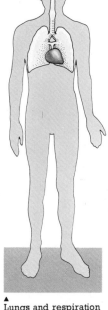

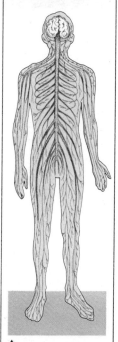

▲
Digestive system

▲
Heart and circulation

▲
Lungs and respiration

▲
Brain: nervous system

The Power Station
When food is eaten, energy extracted by the gut passes into the blood and is stored in the muscles, liver and, as fat, almost anywhere. When air enters the lungs, oxygen is transferred

to the blood. The heart continuously pumps the blood, rich with fuel and oxygen to all parts of the body. When the machine works, the fuel in the blood is burnt with the oxygen, creating

exhaust products (mainly carbondioxide and water) which are carried by the blood back to the lungs. The system operates non-stop throughout life.

The Computer
Information travels through the system in the form of small electrical charges. The sense organs, ears, eyes etc., convert stimuli into these electrical messages.

Balanced diet

Food breaks down basically into fat, protein and carbohydrate, plus very small amounts of various vitamins and minerals, and water. The normal diet of a person in a technological society includes all the vitamins and minerals needed. There is still no completely convincing evidence that extra doses of these are really needed by the sports-man. Since the sportsman sweats a lot, he needs to drink a lot of water, but in normal circumstances his thirst is the best guide as to how much he needs to drink. It is only during unaccustomed exposure to very hot environments, or when needing to lose weight tempo-rarily, that he should take more or less than his thirst dictates.

EXAMPLE	ENERGY Kcals	WATER g	PROTEIN g	FAT g	CARBO-HYDRATE	ALCOHOL %
Bread, white	245	38·0	8·0	1·4	52·0	
Bread, wholemeal	240	41·0	9·0	2·0	47·0	
Flour, white	350	14·0	10·0	1·5	74·0	
Flour, wholewheat	340	15·0	12·0	2·0	71·0	
Rice, white, boiled	103	72·0	2·0	0·2	23·0	
Rice, brown, boiled	115	70·0	2·4	0·5	25·0	
Cornflakes	363	3·0	8·0	1·0	79·0	
Muesli	396	5·0	18·0	2·0	74·0	
Egg (2, whole)	150	66·0	11·0	11·0	1·0	
Bacon, fried	700	13·0	22·0	67·0	2·0	
Beef, minced	260	56·0	20·0	20·0	0	
Beef, steak, grilled	396	47·6	26·0	32·3	0	
Beef, roasted	220	60·0	25·0	13·0	0	
Chicken, roasted	150	62·0	30·0	3·0	0	
Lamb, roasted	350	48·0	20·0	30·0	0	
Lamb, stewed	147	70·6	9·0	8·5	8·0	
Liver, pig, fried	230	54·0	30·0	11·0	2·5	
Turkey, roasted	260	55·0	28·0	15·0	0	
Haddock, fried	175	65·0	20·4	8·3	3·6	

Typical foods

The charts below and on the facing page show the constituents of typical basic foods: per 100g(3.5oz) solids, and 100ml(0.2pt) liquids.

EXAMPLE	ENERGY Kcals	WATER g	PROTEIN g	FAT g	CARBO-HYDRATE	ALCOHOL %
Plaice, fried	140	38·0	11·0	9·0	4·0	
Beans, runner, boiled	41	90·0	1·0	2·0	10·0	
Beans, haricot, baked	110	67·0	6·0	0·5	21·0	
Cabbage, boiled	25	92·0	1·2	0·2	4·0	
Cauliflower, boiled	35	94·0	2·0	0	3·0	
Celery, raw	16	95·0	1·0	0	2·0	
Lettuce (20g)	5	19·0	0·2	0	0·4	
Mushrooms, fried	165	70·0	2·5	15·0	4·0	
Onions, raw	35	90·0	1·5	0	8·0	
Potatoes, boiled	77	80·0	2·0	0·2	18·0	
Apple	55	80·0	0·4	0·3	13·0	
Grapefruit	18	46·0	2·8	0	4·0	
Orange	35	63·0	1·0	0·2	8·0	
Peach	38	81·0	0·5	0	9·0	
Strawberries	40	88·0	0·6	0·4	9·0	
Milk	66	90·0	3·6	3·6	4·8	
Cream, double (25g)	110	12·0	0·4	12·0	0·6	
Butter (25g)	180	3·7	0·2	21·0	0·2	
Cheese, cheddar	400	36·0	26·0	33·5	0·5	
Cheese, cottage	75	75·0	18·0	0·5	0	
Yoghurt, plain	43	76·0	3·6	1·0	5·0	
Sugar, white (20g)	100	0	0	0	20·0	
Sugar, brown (20g)	80	0	0	0	20·0	
Tea, without milk	3	101	0·1	0	0·1	
Coffee, without milk	3	102	0	0	0·3	
Beer, (220ml/0·4pt)	100	212	0·6	0	7·0	4
Spirits (70° proof)	210	64	0	0	0	32
Wine, red	95	82	0·3	0	0·5	12·5
Wine, white	90	84	0·2	0	4·0	10·0

per 100g (3·5oz) solids and 100ml (0·2pt) liquids

The machine at work

The human is the most uniquely gifted animal, Though individual species can run faster, jump higher, swim faster, climb, tumble, burrow, etc., better than the human – he is the only animal able to do *all* that the others can – except fly.

The people shown here, be they athletes or not, are all specialists, very highly trained to do their own thing. But, like the rest of us, they still have general fitness to some extent – and all of us have the capacity of the human machine. That is, to do any one of these activities, and others, to a very high degree – and to do all of them at a reasonable level.

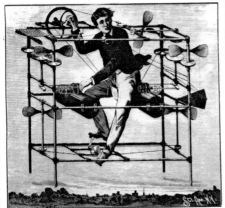

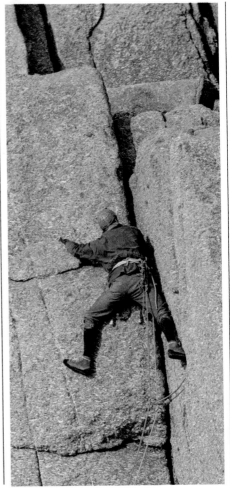

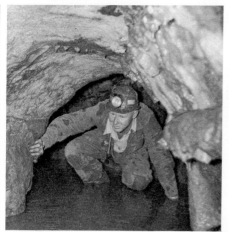

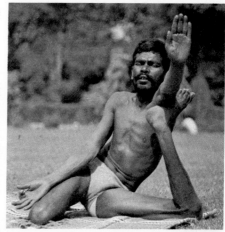

Cliff climbing and potholing are activities which require immense concentration The Indian Yogi, *above right*, achieves these qualities to an extreme degree. Through his spiritual and physical training he is able to assume postures that seem inconceivable.

The flying machine, *far left*, designed by Dr Ayres of New Haven, USA, in 1885 typifies man's ambition to fly, with the aid of a springboard, *right*, he can momentarily capture the grace of a winged creature.

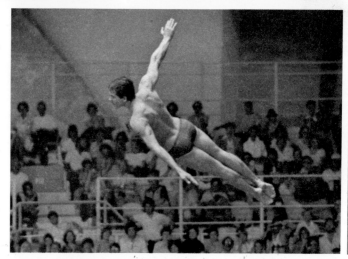

The road to fitness

The road to fitness is called *Progressive Overload*. Almost all human tissues, with the important exception of the brain, respond to progressively increasing loads by progressively increasing their function. The only practical limit to this development seems to be the amount of time, energy and fuel made available. When the machine is given progressive overload, that is called *training*. Without overload, *training* does not occur. With too much overload, strain will occur. The broad road to fitness chosen by each individual must run carefully between too little and too much.

Training, not torture

To most people the word training is equated with torture, and certainly some of the roads to fitness are tortuous! But they need not be. Other roads are simple, pleasant and safe – and get you there just as quickly. It is easier to consider training as an effect, a benefit gained from following a programme of enjoyable activities. With this approach, although the initial reason for undertaking the activities is to achieve fitness, the activities soon become so enjoyable that they are done for their own sake. Most people are easily diverted from the road to fitness quite soon after starting their journey. When the road is enjoyable for its own sake – drop outs are rare!

TERMINOLOGY

There are some specialist terms used in training:

A Repetition – one complete exercise (sometimes abbreviated to 'rep')

A Set – a number of reps of the same exercise without stopping

A Series – a number of sets, with a rest between each

A Session – a number of series of different or similar exercises

Cheating – altering an exercise slightly to make it easier

Load – the amount of resistance to an exercise

Physical activities

PAP

This is your Physical Activities Programme. It is personal to you, and designed by you. Together with your social activities, your work activities and your cultural activities programmes, it makes up almost all of your waking life. It may indeed combine with them, even to the extent that work, social and physical activities can sometimes all be done together.

In most cases each individual's PAP will be designed by himself. He needs good advice, some of which will be provided by this book. Other sources of advice are sports coaches, physical educators, physiotherapists and similar professions.

When setting off along this road, it is essential to make sure that the machine doesn't have any defects which are going to cause a breakdown. Some machines are more likely to have defects than others. If you haven't taken strenuous exercise for a long time, or have a family history of heart disease, or have suffered from serious illness or injury yourself, you should have a thorough medical checkup before starting.

PREPARATION

The latter sections of this book tell you how to prepare your own PAP, but its effectiveness will depend on some general preparations which you should always make, and check, before starting each and every session of activity. These are POCKETS.

P – place of activities; have you booked it, will it be open?

O – other people involved; do they know, are they organised?

C – content; have you planned the content of your session to fit PAP?

K – Kit; is everything in your bag, is it serviceable?

E – equipment; is it available, suitable, prepared, serviceable?

T – time; are you sure of the time and likely duration of the session?

S – safety; are you using the right equipment, methods, precautions?

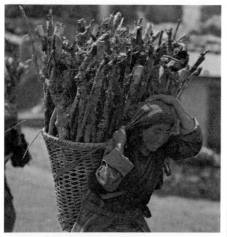

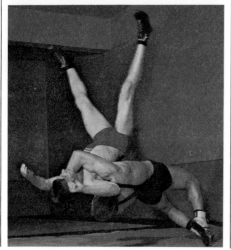

Strength

Muscles can become stronger in two major ways: by increasing quantity and quality. Bigger muscles are usually stronger muscles, so quantity of muscle is important. It is also possible to increase muscle strength without increasing the overall size of the muscle, that is, to increase its quality. But some people want bigger muscles in order to look good, and in this case quality of muscle is not of such great importance.

Resistance

When resistance to the muscles is great, movement may be slow, may not occur at all, or may be overcome and move in the opposite direction. These movements are called *concentric, static* and *eccentric*. The methods of increasing strength all involve working the muscles against resistance. By steadily increasing the load, and the number of repetitions, the muscle gets bigger and stronger. There are many forms of resistance, including your own body, a partner, weights, springs, elastic materials, and machines. Static exercises involving the trunk should not be performed, particularly while holding the breath, since thereby great pressure is built up inside the chest which hampers the function of the heart.

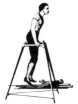

Strength and big muscles do not always go together. The Sherpa woman carrying a huge load looks almost frail, but the weight seems to give her no trouble. Wrestling, *below left*, is a sport in which quality of muscle is needed to maintain speed with strength. Bodybuilders, *right*, invariably have the biggest muscles but not necessarily the highest quality. A hammer thrower or weightlifter, for example, would certainly be able to produce more power.

Below
A demonstration of the overload principle!

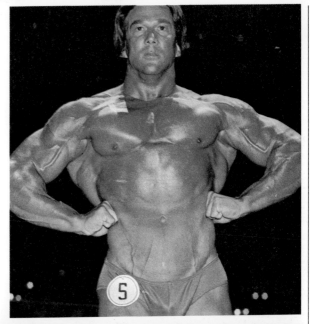

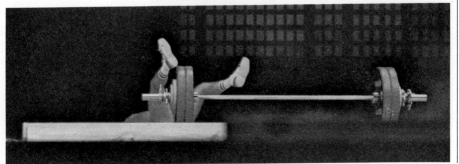

Speed

Speed comprises two main elements: response to a stimulus, and high velocity.

Stimulus – response (S-R)

This in itself divides into several sections:

1. Detection of the stimulus (receiving information)
2. Analysis and decision making (processing information)
3. Initiating the response (sending information)

Since information can only travel along the nerves at a pre-set rate, there is not much that a normal healthy person can do to improve the rate. Pure reflex actions (such as the knee jerk reflex tested by the doctor) cannot be speeded up by training, though they can deteriorate in ill health.

But in more complex S-R situations you can certainly learn to speed things up, by improving your ability to detect relevant information, and to process that information.

Detection

To improve this, you need to learn how to spot relevant information amongst the mass of information confronting you. For example, if whilst driving you learn always to look through the windows of the car in front, you will spot emergencies before the brake lights of that car give you the usual signal to slow down. A good games player will look for early hints by his opponent as to what he is going to do, thus giving himself more time to respond.

Processing

By learning a series of responses to fairly standard situations, it is possible to do away with the analysis part of the S-R completely. It is also useful to develop techniques of analysing information, rather than random thought processes, so that thinking time can also be cut down.

The secret of developing S-R speed is highly repetitive practice in an analytical frame of mind, and in some cases ultra highly repetitive practice doing away with the mind altogether!

High velocity

Again the situation is complicated. Is the desired high velocity to be in one part of the body (like the upper limb in piano playing), or the whole body (like sprint running), or in some other object moved by the body (like throwing a javelin)?

Power and weight

Power to Weight Ratio

There is also the effect on speed of the Power to Weight Ratio. The more powerful the person, the higher the speed he can generate. The greater the weight to be moved, the slower the speed. So, if greater power is developed but at the expense of greater weight, the net result is no change in speed.

When you put these two together you find that great speed can be developed in a light limb by a heavy body, the power being transferred from the powerful body to the lighter limb. This is why many good golfers have quite heavy bodies. On the other hand, if the whole body has to be moved, then too much weight is a hindrance. Sprinters tend to be muscular but of medium weight. Finally, if the body's power has to be transferred to another object, it pays to be very big and powerful – like the shot putter.

Apart from these specialist examples, it is clear that Mr. Average needs to reduce his nonproductive weight (fat), and increase his strength and muscularity to a reasonable degree, in order to be able to generate high velocity.

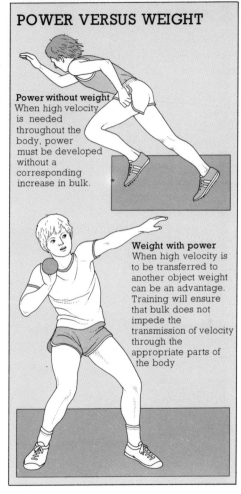

POWER VERSUS WEIGHT

Power without weight
When high velocity is needed throughout the body, power must be developed without a corresponding increase in bulk.

Weight with power
When high velocity is to be transferred to another object weight can be an advantage. Training will ensure that bulk does not impede the transmission of velocity through the appropriate parts of the body

Stamina

By now, the reader will have realised that no fitness element is simple. Stamina is no exception, even though it may be defined simply as 'the ability to keep going'. Stamina can involve withstanding the feelings of fatigue – or not getting the feelings at all! Fatigue includes the actual 'chemical' state of muscles, and the feelings which accompany that state. Stamina is needed to work for many hours at a light task, or to repeat a very heavy action.

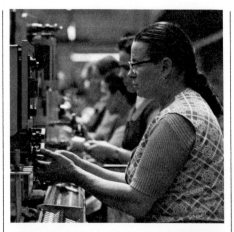

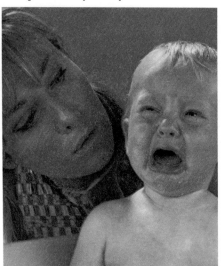

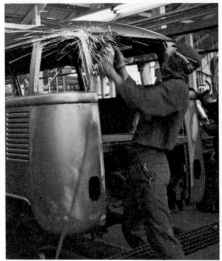

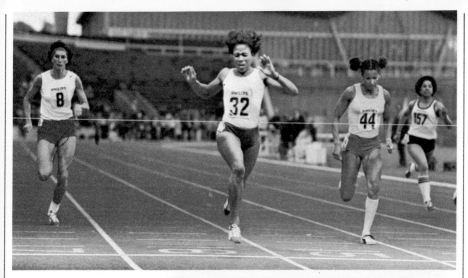

There are many non-sporting activities for which stamina is needed. Whether at the factory bench, on the workshop floor, felling trees or coping with a demanding child, stamina is required in order to keep going. In all prolonged, repetitive activities, muscle stamina is necessary to sustain the action. Even short-distance runners, *above*, make many repetitions of the same action. In running, stamina is not just a matter of being able to run for hours, it is also part of being able to cover a distance at competitive speed.

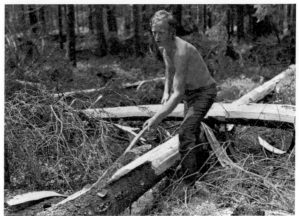

Developing stamina

Let us look at the various parts of the machine, and get an idea of how to develop stamina in each.

Muscle stamina

Since muscle stores its own fuel, its stamina is determined by its ability to hold large stores, and its efficiency at processing these in terms of taking fuel out of the blood, and getting rid of the waste products of consuming that fuel.

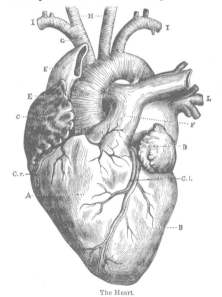

The Heart.

This facility is developed by performing very high numbers of repetitions of actions. Quite literally, hundreds of thousands of repetitions, in large sets. For example, a marathon runner may take over 20,000 strides in one training session.

Circulation

Since the heart never stops beating, it demonstrates stamina *par excellence*! But, there are times when it is required to increase its output by as much as sixfold. Its abilities to work for long periods at high rates, and to recover quickly from such activity, are the two major factors in developing circulatory fitness.

It is virtually impossible to strain the healthy heart, and overload training for the heart is best achieved by very heavy exercise maintained for medium time periods – between a minute and twenty minutes. 'Circuit Training' is the most effective way of doing this. At the level of sedentary man, activities must produce a heart rate at least equal to that given by the simple formula shown on the opposite page,★ if they are to produce a training effect.

For a superfit athlete, somewhat higher rates are needed. Heart rate should be measured immediately exercise stops, by clamping the hand both sides of the throat under the chin. The pulse will be felt clearly. The number of beats in 10 seconds should be counted, then multiplied by 6 to give the heart rate.

Circulatory recovery training is achieved by 'Interval Training', of which there are several types. The idea is to exercise flat out for a short time (between 15 seconds and a few minutes) several times, with short rest intervals between.

Mind

Since most of the things which cause you to stop activity when fatigued are sensations of the mind, it is possible to improve stamina enormously by training the mind firstly to be less aware of fatigue, and secondly to fight through it even when it does intrude into the mind. This is achieved by repeated overload exposure of the mind to fatigue of all kinds which allows mental acclimatisation to take place; and further by mental distraction exercises during fatigue, especially those which concentrate on some other aim of the physical activity – such as winning!

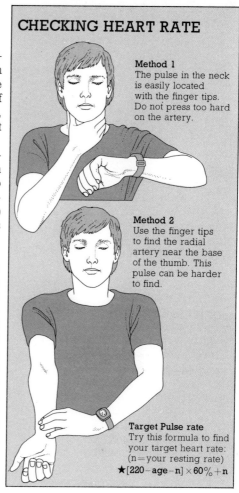

CHECKING HEART RATE

Method 1
The pulse in the neck is easily located with the finger tips. Do not press too hard on the artery.

Method 2
Use the finger tips to find the radial artery near the base of the thumb. This pulse can be harder to find.

Target Pulse rate
Try this formula to find your target heart rate:
(n = your resting rate)
$\star [220 - \text{age} - \text{n}] \times 60\% + \text{n}$

Suppleness

Suppleness depends upon the elasticity of muscles, and the range of movement possible at the joints. You can test the former when touching your toes with your knees straight. The resulting tightness at the rear of the thigh is because the hamstring muscles are insufficiently elastic. Joint movement is restricted either by the shape of the bones (like when you try to straighten your elbow too far) or by the tightness of the ligaments holding the joint together.

Ligament stretching

This is a much longer process, accomplished by manipulating the joint to stretch the ligaments concerned. It is much more difficult to tear a ligament than a muscle, and more force can be used; but the same care needs to be used by you, or your helpers.

With persistence, phenomenal degrees of suppleness *can* be achieved, especially in young people where a certain degree of 'bone moulding' can also take place. But, there has to be a reason for the suppleness. Too much is usually more dangerous than too little. Many first-class athletes concentrate on muscle rather than ligament stretching in their exercise programmes.

MUSCLE STRETCHING

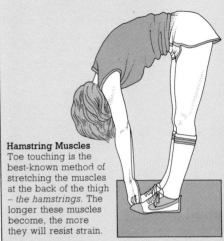

Hamstring Muscles
Toe touching is the best-known method of stretching the muscles at the back of the thigh – *the hamstrings*. The longer these muscles become, the more they will resist strain.

Muscle lengths can quite easily be altered by training. After warming up with some general activity, the muscle must gradually be stretched by movement at the surrounding joints. This can be a dangerous process since, if too violent, it can lead to muscle tears. The safest method is to do the movements under your own steam, stretching the muscle to the limit of discomfort, but not so as to cause pain. It is also possible to accomplish good results with a skilled person stretching the muscle by manipulating the bones.

Skill

Skill borrows a little from the other fitness elements. If you are not strong, then some actions will cause you to strain hard instead of maintaining an easy control. Similarly, a lack of speed and stamina makes skill difficult to achieve.

The first part of skill is concerned with making the right decisions, which we covered in the section on speed. The action messages are then transmitted to muscles, which perform the actions required. Once the body knows what it has to do, knows the right decisions, practise of the action is rather like a stream trickling down hill. With many repetitions the stream will find the easiest way down hill, and groove itself so deeply into the ground that it becomes smooth and clear forever. Occasionally, a water engineer might spot a slight improvement, and change the course of the stream. Similarly, a good teacher can spot faults creeping into skilled action, and correct them before they become too grooved. These skills, called *closed skills*, are the most efficient because once the decision to do them has been made, no more thought is necessary, like changing gear, using cutlery, etc.

Open skills

These are much more difficult, when the conditions are not identical every time, and you have to work out a unique physical action just for that one occasion. In this case, it helps if you have a wide variety of little 'closed' skills at your disposal which you can perform very effectively. All you need to do then is to string all the most suitable ones together to make the total action. This ability is developed by practising many different skills in a constantly changing situation. Playing soccer is rather like that.

Skills should be practised little and often, not practising in a fatigued condition *until* the skill is well learned. Accuracy is more important than speed in the early stages, though practice should always be at the highest speed at which accuracy can be maintained.

Open skills
Soccer is a good example of a game in which the player needs to have a variety of skills at his disposal. He will be presented with many 'new' situations in rapid sequence and must respond quickly with the correct skill.

35

The danger zones

Though poor fitness gradually attacks the whole of the body, there are some *Danger Zones* which are most affected. These show up earliest, and perform the useful function of 'early warning signals'. By regularly giving yourself a simple checkup, you can be sure to spot danger signals. This gives you the chance of taking remedial action before the condition begins to accelerate.

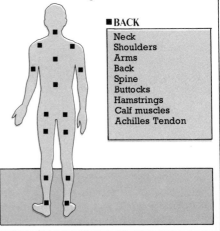

● FRONT

Eyes
Chest
Arms
Stomach
Fingers
Thighs
Groin
Knees
Ankles
Feet

■ BACK

Neck
Shoulders
Arms
Back
Spine
Buttocks
Hamstrings
Calf muscles
Achilles Tendon

BODY AREA	DANGER SIGNAL
Eyes	Tired, sore, aching
Chest	Pains, stitch, short winded
Stomach	Fat fold, distension
Arms	Elbow pains, finger pains
Groin	Strain, hernia
Thighs	Fat fold
Knees	Cartilage, knee cap pains
Ankles	Strains
Feet	Arch pains, bunions, toe pains

BODY ZONE	DANGER SIGNAL
Neck	Muscle pains, posture
Shoulders	Pains, posture
Back	Fat folds
Spine	Disc spots, strains
Arms	Fat folds
Buttocks	Fat folds
Hamstring	Strains
Calf	Varicose veins
Achilles Tendon	Tendonitis, inflammation pains

Warming up

We keep thinking of the human as a machine, and like a machine he gets hot when he works. The fuel and oxygen may not actually explode in his tissues, but heat is produced not only where the fuel is consumed, but also by the small amount of friction in the various moving parts. Just like a car engine, the human is more efficient when warmed up, and less likely to suffer damage. In fact, the internal temperature of marathon runners can be higher than the temperature which would kill a man suffering a high fever.

So, it is good common sense to warm up before running the machine hard. You should wear warm clothes and gradually increase the pace of the warm up activities over a period of 5-10 minutes until you are working quite hard. This should be done immediately before the activity you are preparing for, since as soon as you stop warming up – you start cooling down! Particularly with some organs, like heart and lungs, recovery can be complete within a minute or two.

Warming up should involve some stretching of muscles and joints which are required to be mobile, and gross movements like running or jumping.

WARMING DOWN

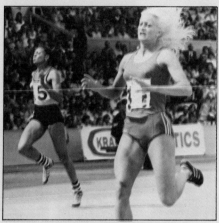

This is the bit almost everyone forgets. But in fact the scientific reasons for warm down are stronger than those for warm up. Recovery after exercise is assisted greatly by keeping the machine ticking over at a gentle rate. Particularly, the movement of limbs helps the blood back to the heart by massaging the veins. This helps to eliminate waste products, and replenish fuel supplies in the muscles.

Again, the body should be protected against too rapid cooling of the skin, by wearing loose clothing.

Strength programmes

It is important to realise that most muscle groups are balanced by other groups performing an opposite action – called *antagonists*. The balance between these is of enormous importance. Work done in developing the one must be linked with work on the antagonists.

Normally, one side of the body is much stronger than the other, but this is a developed state. Our natural state is to be almost equally balanced. Any imbalance tends to cause bad posture, itself leading to arthritis, slipped disc and other problems. Strength training produces a balanced development.

In this programme we are just concerned with the muscles of the body. Since there are 215 pairs of them, it is easier to deal with them in groups by their location and their function.

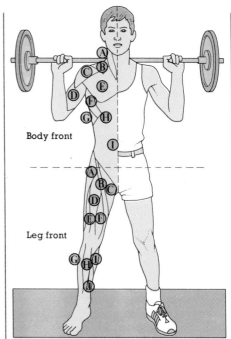

Body front

Leg front

BODY FRONT	
A	Sternomastoid
B	Trapezius
C	Deltoid
D	Biceps
E	Pectoralis
F	Serratus
G	Latissimus
H	External Oblique
I	Rectus Abdominis

LEG FRONT	
A	Tensor Fasciae Latae
B	Sartorius
C	Adductors
D	Rectus Femoris of Quadriceps
E	Outer Head of Quadriceps
F	Inner Head of Quadriceps
G	Peronei
H	Anterior Tibial Muscle
I	Inner edge of Gastrocnemus
J	Inner edge of Soleus

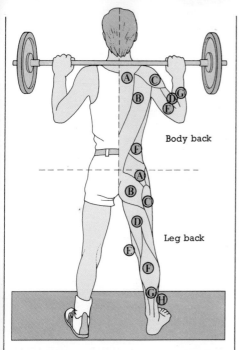

Body back

Leg back

Muscle structure

The diagrams on the left show the general position of the muscles we are concerned with, their correct anatomical names being listed in the charts beneath.

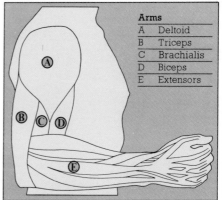

Arms	
A	Deltoid
B	Triceps
C	Brachialis
D	Biceps
E	Extensors

BODY BACK	
A	Trapezius
B	Latissimus
C	Deltoid
D	Biceps
E	Triceps
F	External oblique
G	Flexors and Extensors

LEG BACK	
A	Gluteus Medius
B	Gluteus Maximus
C	Tensor Fasciae Latae
D	Hamstrings
E	Sartorius
F	Gastrocnemius
G	Soleus
H	Peronei

Strength clothing

Strength training is not continuous work. There is more time spent resting than there is working. If the room temperature is cold, warm clothing should be worn in order to keep the body temperature high, but should be loose so that movement is not restricted.

Strong movements put great stress on various body parts. Correct clothing can reduce the effects of this stress. Starting with the feet, which take all the weight and shock, it is advisable to wear flat soled shoes with a reasonable internal arch support. Extra support is gained by using high cut shoes (boots) extending an inch or two above the ankles. Comfortable socks should be worn.

Except for deep knee movements in competitive weightlifting, knee bandages should not be used.

It is advisable for male genitalia and female breasts to be firmly supported, and persons performing strong movements above the head with the back arched should wear a broad supporting belt.

If weights are to be carried on body parts other than the hands, protective padding should be used to avoid bruising, like a folded towel on shoulders.

Weightlifting dress
The most important item is the broad supporting belt around the abdomen and lower back.

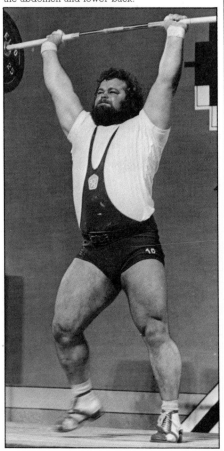

Strength safety

Any strength training which increases the forces passing through the body poses its own dangers. Body tissues can be torn, bruised and fractured so very easily. Great care and control are necessary, and it is advisable to have someone else present when exercising who can help when an exercise may be going wrong. Also, it is common to have safety built into machines and resistance systems so that if the body collapses some other structure can take the strain. But common sense and foresight are the most important aids.

Another problem is the sheer wear and tear on the joints, with all the extra weight passing through the 'bearings'. Up to a certain level (which is impossible to measure accurately) this extra stimulus develops the articulating surfaces. But over and above these loads, the joint surfaces gradually break down and wear away – leading to arthritic changes in some cases. It is possible to have too much of this particular good thing. In general, if you can so position yourself that the resistance is tending to pull a joint apart rather than compress it you will reduce this wear.

SAFETY HINTS

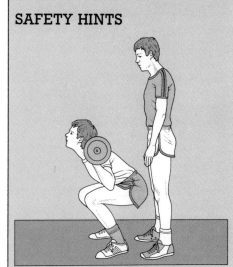

Exercising joints beyond their 'non return' point is dangerous, since the mechanical disadvantages thus created exaggerate the wear forces. For example, heavy 'squatting' exercises ought not to go beyond 90° at the knees, and trunk flexing whilst carrying heavy weights ought not to go beyond a similar angle.
The problem with this exercise is that on the last repetition you might not make it, in which case you need a human catcher. Don't try it without one; it is potentially dangerous.

41

Bodyweight exercises

In performing bodyweight exercises, as the term implies, you rely on your own weight to provide the necessary resistance. Although some gymnasium equipment, such as beams and wall bars, may be helpful many of these exercises can be done at home without any special equipment. As a means of developing bodily strength without undue increase in bulk they are ideal. With ingenuity you can invent many other similar exercises, but remember, for strength training they must be hard.

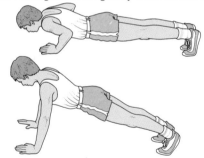

Arm & shoulder extend
Good old pressups are still the best. To increase the resistance raise the feet on a box or table; to lower it, rest the hands on a box or table. Keep the body straight, and only the nose should touch the floor.

ARM AND SHOULDER

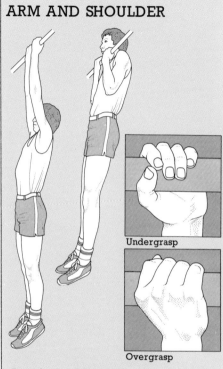

Undergrasp

Overgrasp

Arm & shoulder flex
Using sometimes an overgrasp and sometimes an undergrasp, smoothly pull up to touch the bar with the chin. If too weak to do the movement, try resting your feet on a stool or table to reduce the resistance.

TRUNK

Bodyweight exercises

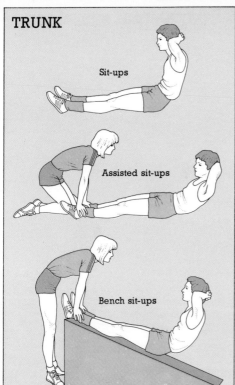

Sit-ups

Assisted sit-ups

Bench sit-ups

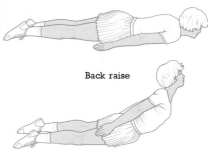

Back raise

Trunk extend
This always seems an awkward exercise to perform, but it is very useful for protecting the spine against disc problems and back strains.

Trunk flex
Sit-ups, another old favourite. Don't pull on the neck. Secure the feet to make it easier. To make it harder, lie feet high on an incline – until you can do them hanging upside down.

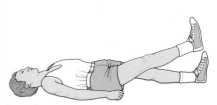

Leg flex
This exercise is generally neglected, but is still important. Take the movement as far as you can, and hold it in the extreme position by tensing the muscles hard for a few seconds.

43

LEGS AND ANKLES

Bodyweight exercises

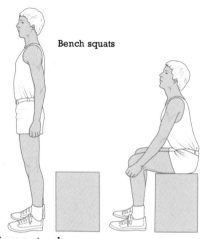

Bench squats

Ankle extend

Heel raises with the toes on a block or step, touching a wall or prop in order to maintain balance. Get as big a range of movement as possible and move explosively. If too easy, do them one leg at a time.

Ankle flex

Putting one heel on the toes of the working leg lift the foot slowly, leaving its heel on the ground, against the resistance of the weight of the other leg. Use a full range of movement.

Ankle flex

Leg extend

There are many varieties of squats, but bench squats are the safest,– the knee doesn't bend too far. If the exercise is too easy, do it with one leg at a time – but smoothly.

Barbell exercises

The use of weights allows exercises to be designed far more precisely than bodyweight can. Consequently, the range of exercises is very great, and only a representative sample can be shown here.

Load

For high quality of muscle, loads must be very high, permitting only one or two repetitions to be performed. For large muscle bulk, lower loads and more repetitions (up to about 10) are better. A well balanced series will start with low loads/high repetitions, working up to high loads/low repetitions, and then perhaps back again. Do a maximum of 3 sets × 10 repetitions of each exercise. If 10 are too easy then increase the resistance.

Weight training is of considerable benefit to most sportsmen and women. High repetitions with weights will make a significant contribution to any stamina programme because they will help to increase endurance for the stamina training. Indeed, there are few sports in which improved strength is not beneficial. Women should not be afraid of weight training: big muscle development requires the presence of male hormones.

FOREARM AND BICEPS

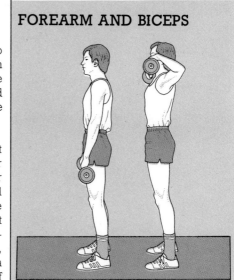

Elbow flex
Particularly good for forearm and the famous biceps muscle. It helps if, when at the midway sticking point on the last repetitions, you cheat a little by swaying your upper body. Occasionally change from under to over grasp.

Barbell exercises

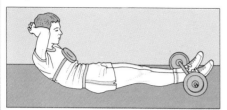

◄ *Abdominal flex*
The sit up exercise is much more powerful with the feet secured and weight disc carried on the chest. The exercise is better done on a mat, to avoid bruising the back. The weights should rest on chest muscle.

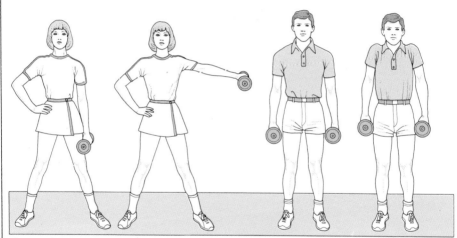

Arm raise
This exercise can be done with one arm, or both simultaneously, and with under and over grip. With one arm, try to keep the upper body erect. This is one of the best exercises for improving shoulder strength.

Shoulder raise
In this case, the neck muscles are being worked, giving sloping shoulders and a bigger neck. The exercise is, quite simply, a shrug of the shoulders against resistance.

Barbell exercises

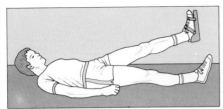

◄ **Leg flex**
This exercise needs the 'iron boot' since it is the only reasonable way of applying the resistance. Not much weight is needed since it is a very hard exercise, but a very good one. Lower the weight slowly.

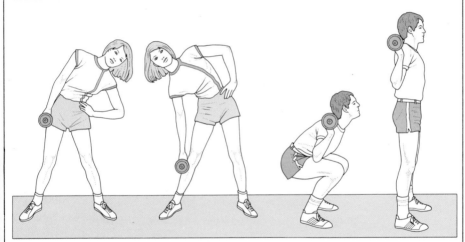

Trunk side bends
Another frequently neglected exercise, the muscles on the side opposite the weight being the ones exercised. Use a full range of movement, and it becomes a suppleness exercise as well.

Leg extend
Heavy squats are a favourite exercise, but should only go as far as 90°. The bar should be taken from and replaced on a rack, or helpers' hands. Keep the back straight during the whole of this exercise.

Barbell exercises

Elbow extend
This should be performed in conjunction with the biceps exercise shown on page 45. In this, the antagonist triceps muscle is worked on, using the same principle. Without balanced development of triceps, the arms tend to hang in crooked 'ape' like fashion.

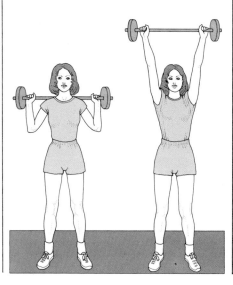

'MAKE DO' EXERCISES

There are, of course, many other forms of resistance (springs, rubber, hydraulic, magnetic, etc.) What is probably more important is that quite ordinary objects around the house or works can be used for strength training.

Wrist rolling
A 2" diameter stick, 3' of strong cord and a house brick make a fine forearm exercise machine. By winding the brick up and down, then reversing from over to under grip, superb forearms can be developed.

Chest and shoulder Exercise
Two old flat irons, weighted handbags, large tins filled with sand etc., make fine barbells for this superb exercise.

Make exercise enjoyable
Strength activities are the most difficult to make enjoyable. Introducing an element of competition can help – such as 'arm wrestling' – but it is often possible to do ordinary work or domestic tasks in such a way that they become good strength exercises. With ingenuity almost any lifting job can be a maximum exercise for some part of the body.

Exercise machines

There is a variety of exercise machines available these days in well equipped clubs and centres. Some are multi-station machines such as the *Ergogym*. Others are single station specialist machines.

The squat machine permits very safe squatting; *the 'Lats' machine* is excellent for developing the 'triangular' look; *Pulley systems* are excellent for getting the right direction of move-ment. *The Quadriceps machine* allows very heavy leg exercise to be performed without carrying heavy weights on the shoulders, and without heavy wearing stresses going through the knee joint.

The multistation machine shown here, with its pulley systems, weights, benches and fixed positions, reproduces many of the elements contained in the strength programme.

Bodyweight exercises

1. sit-ups
2. sit-ups
3. elbow flex – chins
4. dips

Simulated barbell exercises

5. leg press
6. bench press
7. spring pulley
8. rowing pulley
9. elbow flex

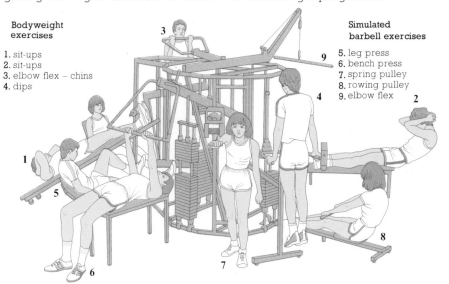

Speed programmes

Speed training covers the stimulus-response mechanism, and the high velocity mechanism. In both cases the body requires the use of strong quick muscles and what we call *levers*. Various parts of the body actually form levers. The way in which these levers are used can favour speed at the expense of force, or vice versa. Muscles can be made stronger, but also intrinsically faster, by altering the balance of fast and slow fibres in the muscle. Stronger and faster means more powerful.

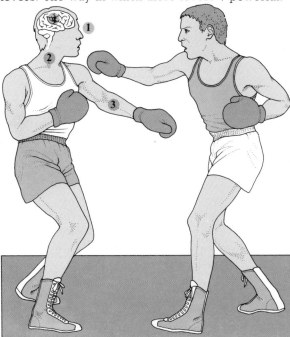

Stimulus – Response (SR)

SR is not so complicated as it sounds. A simple breakdown of a typical punch and counter-punch action in the boxing ring will explain how it works.

1st response:

The stimulus of an approaching glove will tend to cause a reflex blink of the eyes.

2nd response:

The brain instructs the neck muscles to shift the head out of the path of the approaching blow.

3rd response:

The brain decides that the blow should be parried and sends action messages to the arm.

4th response:

The brain evaluates the potential effect of a counter punch and instructs the muscles to effect the action.

Levers

Long levers

The discus thrower uses a long lever – a fully extended arm – to generate high velocity at the extreme end of the lever. This speed is passed directly to the implement. With a correct angle of elevation, the discus will reach a considerable height and still have much of its forward velocity during its descent.

Short levers

The wrestler adopts short levers for strength and quick responses. Bent arms can make short, sharp movements which exert considerable power and yet remain under control. The wrestler is thereby able to adjust quickly to the changing situation and is always ready to shift his weight and strength into a new position.

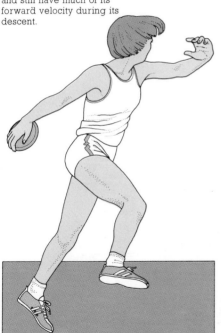

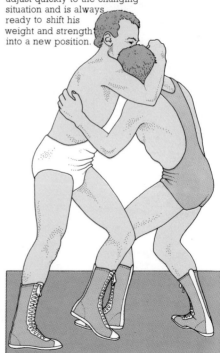

The levers

Many people get very confused about the use of levers. On one hand, where the resistance to speed is rather small, long levers develop high velocity at the end of the lever. So golfers, racquet players and fly swatters use long limbs and implements. Where the resistance is proportionally greater and/or response speed is more important than high velocity, short levers are frequently used, such as boxing (particularly the uppercut), and slip fielding at cricket.

The principle can be seen clearly in using a shovel. If high velocity is needed to be developed in the contents of the shovel, to throw them a long distance, the arms should be extended and the movement generated almost entirely from the trunk and legs. On the other hand, to shift soil quickly into a nearby barrow, bent arm movements using more shoulder and arm muscles is more effective.

When training for speed, analyse what kind of levers suit the purpose best, and develop that skill and those muscles by repetition training.

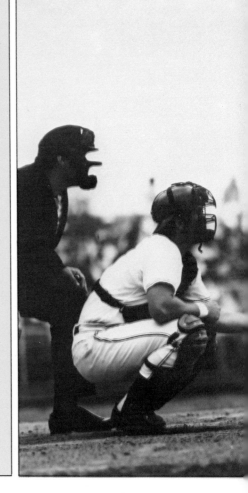

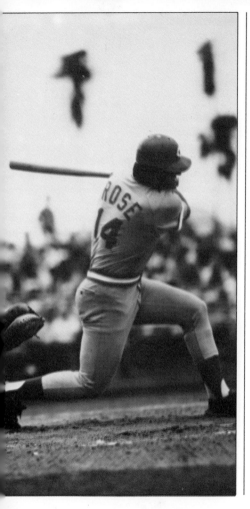

Speed is everywhere

Most people think fast movements are only for superfit performers like sportsmen and dancers. not so – life is short, and the quicker we can do some things the more time we have to spare for others. Most of the routine actions we perform in life can be speeded up without ill effects and with many benefits. The attempt to make movements quicker will often ensure that we use a a more efficient action, for example brushing teeth and cleaning windows.

Become speed minded. When you walk between rooms, walk quickly: climb stairs at a run, but one at a time so that the feet move more quickly: deal the cards for bridge more quickly: train yourself in fast reading and speed-writing.

The net result of this will be more time to linger over the things you really enjoy – or to try some new activities altogether.

Levers in action
In baseball, the batter tries to inject very high velocity into the ball. He uses the bat as an extension of his arm – lengthening the lever and increasing the speed of impact. The catcher uses his arm as a short lever for quick responses.

Speed clothing

When training the reception of information, clothing can act as resistance which overloads the receptors concerned, thus developing them. Wearing sunglasses can reduce visual signals, ear muffs can reduce sound, and gloves can reduce tactile and pressure reception. If some training is undertaken wearing such clothing, with a conscious concentration on the detection of the information concerned, there will be an improvement in performance.

When working on the speed of muscle actions, sufficient clothing should be worn to keep the muscles warm, but of a light and unrestrictive form so that the movements are not hampered.

Since high velocity movements are generally powerful ones, it is important that good traction is obtained with any adjoining surfaces. Shoes therefore should have a good adhesive tread or studs, in order to prevent slipping.

Speed training also can involve very sudden jerky movements which may endanger male genitalia and female breasts. Good supporting clothing ought to be worn in these situations.

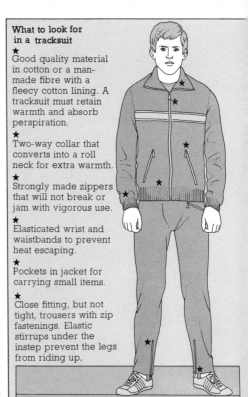

What to look for in a tracksuit

★ Good quality material in cotton or a man-made fibre with a fleecy cotton lining. A tracksuit must retain warmth and absorb perspiration.

★ Two-way collar that converts into a roll neck for extra warmth.

★ Strongly made zippers that will not break or jam with vigorous use.

★ Elasticated wrist and waistbands to prevent heat escaping.

★ Pockets in jacket for carrying small items.

★ Close fitting, but not tight, trousers with zip fastenings. Elastic stirrups under the instep prevent the legs from riding up,

A well-designed tracksuit is an essential item for most fitness programmes. Its principal benefit comes during warm up and warm down periods, but it also provides a functional outfit for travelling to and from the place of activity.

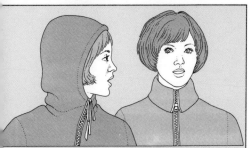

Speed safety

S-R movements tend to be sudden accelerations from resting positions, or sudden changes of direction when already moving. Various massive body parts then behave rather like the standing passenger in a bus doing a sudden stop. They tend to move in the opposite direction to their supporting structures – which can lead to torn fibres and even fractures.

Additionally, high velocity movements occasionally have to stop suddenly. If the buffer which stops them is a ligament, muscle or bone, damage can occur. Tennis elbow is a good example of this, and also bruised heels from jumping.

You should consider the movements you are to perform, and decide if such strains are likely to occur. If so, a slight change in movement, or some material protection, can be very valuable. If it is not possible to achieve protection, then you should always be on the alert to detect early warnings of strain (particularly pains in joints), so that you can stop the activity before the strain becomes chronic. Many people try to train on in spite of the pain from injury. Resist this temptation; the consequences can be serious.

Hooded tops
They keep the head and ears warm in severe weather without restricting activity.

Roll Necks
The most popular form of tracksuit collar amongst athletes. It unzips to form a conventional collar.

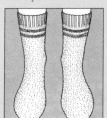

Sports Socks
Good quality absorbant socks are essential. Natural fibres are best. Today, tube socks are becoming popular. They have no heel or toe shaping to form chafing ridges. *See page 64 for shoes.*

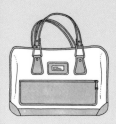

Sports Bag
Look for a good sized 'holdall' for carrying kit, preferably with a separate compartment for muddy footwear. The bag should be as light as possible and have durable handles. Strong zips and locks are essential.

Stimulus response (S-R)

Detection
The receptor organ (ear, eyes, hand, etc.) must be trained to focus on the anticipated source of the signal. Learn to gaze unblinkingly at the approaching fast bowler or the green traffic light, or to touch your opponent (if allowed!) to get an early warning of his movement when you can't see him.

Selection
Train yourself by repeated practice at identifying the important signals from a mass of detail.

Analysis
You must get practice at analysing increasingly complex situations. Look for major points first, then the minor points which refine the situation.

Decision making
Any completely new situation demands a new decision. But with repeated situations you can build up a stock of ready made decisions, so that all you have to do is select the right one once you have analysed the situation.

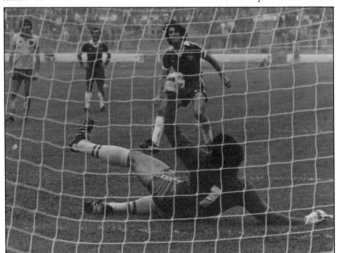

S-R in action
A goalkeeper facing a penalty kick has only a few seconds to analyse the situation and choose his decision from 'stock'. By the time the ball is in the air, the 'keeper will be committed and unable to change his mind. In this case the goalkeeper, diving to his right, is beaten by a ball rising high to his left. This was the result of an incorrect analysis.

S-R training

S-R training can be great fun. Children have invented hundreds of physical games over the years which demand only a small movement, but a very quick decision. These may be simple games such as 'wrist slapping', 'stick catching', or more complicated ones like 'knee boxing', 'Mr Wolf', 'Snap'.

The technological age has swung to the other extreme and provided a huge variety of video games which are superb training devices for S-R ability, like 'Tennis' and 'Shoot Out'.

One great advantage of these is that you can even train by yourself, since the machine can provide you with random stimuli – whereas it is difficult to give these to yourself without a machine.

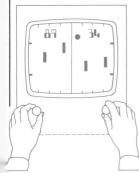

Video games
Simulated tennis, table tennis and soccer video games make good stimulus-response exercises. They first became popular in bars and clubs. Today, many people have them at home.

STIMULUS/RESPONSE GAMES

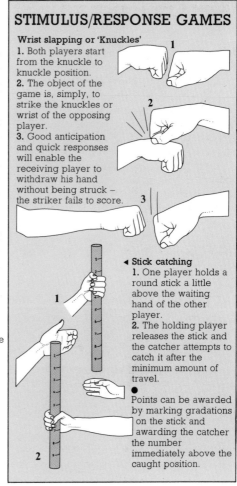

Wrist slapping or 'Knuckles'
1. Both players start from the knuckle to knuckle position.
2. The object of the game is, simply, to strike the knuckles or wrist of the opposing player.
3. Good anticipation and quick responses will enable the receiving player to withdraw his hand without being struck – the striker fails to score.

◄ **Stick catching**
1. One player holds a round stick a little above the waiting hand of the other player.
2. The holding player releases the stick and the catcher attempts to catch it after the minimum amount of travel.

● Points can be awarded by marking gradations on the stick and awarding the catcher the number immediately above the caught position.

Speed training

In most cases, speed can be developed by performing the actions for which speed is required. Runners, cyclists and swimmers all increase the pace of their performances by running, cycling or swimming in training – but not necessarily at racing speeds. As in all forms of training, resistance plays a significant part in speed development, but this is the one programme in which lower resistance is also valuable.

Cyclists and runners can condition their muscle fibres to faster performance by cycling or running, flat out, downhill. The absence of normal resistance may result in faster than racing speeds.

Everybody has two kinds of muscle fibre. For the purposes of training we can call them 'fast' and 'slow' fibres. The purpose of speed training is to develop and condition the fast fibres. The extent to which people can do this varies enormously, but the important factor in speed events is that muscles which have not been introduced, in training, to the speed at which they are require to perform, will not be able to compete at that speed. High velocity training builds the raw ingredient, speed.

SPRINT TRAINING

Sprint cycling
A cyclist has a choice of resistances. He can work uphill for increased resistance, downhill for lower resistance or, for maximum resistance, flat out in low gear.

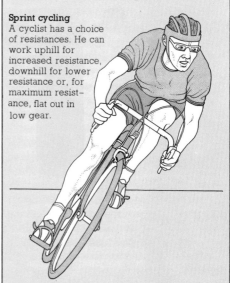

The muscles
Speed is developed by moving very fast. Especially if high velocity needs to be achieved against some resistance, training flat out against a lower resistance helps the fast muscle fibres to develop. These 'sprints' should only be of short duration, perhaps even only one repetition in the set. The set, however, should be repeated several times.

CONCENTRATION

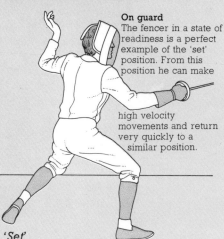

On guard
The fencer in a state of readiness is a perfect example of the 'set' position. From this position he can make high velocity movements and return very quickly to a similar position.

'Set'

In many situations the S-R and muscle systems combine in developing a set state from which a very quick and powerful response can be made. This is a peculiar combination of intense mental concentration, together with a great relaxation of the muscles antagonist to the action to be performed, and a state of preparedness of the muscles which are going to do the work. It must be practised many times, almost to the stage where the stimulus can be anticipated telepathically.

Training against load

Resistance

The muscles: If fast movements have to be performed against much resistance, then great power is needed. Training in this case needs to be against overload, but never such a heavy load that the action becomes ponderous. Speed is still the essence, and it is important that the same style of movement is maintained. There is no point in becoming more powerful but less skilful!

Sprint running
The harness is one of the best methods of resistance sprinting. It is valuable exercise for many sports needing speed.

59

Speed games

If fitness training is to be fun, then games must be the best way of doing it. Here are some games which develop speed of response and high velocity:

●
Table tennis
Excellent for S-R and high speed arm movements and easy to set up in the home or at work. Squash and badminton are less good for S-R, but do use fast whole body actions more.

●
Karate
In playing karate there is a great emphasis on the mental function, as well as the physical actions which are all very fast. Other combat sports are also good for speed training (boxing, fencing, judo, etc.).

●
Basketball
This, the world's most popular ball game, is the best for speed training since it includes exceedingly complex S-R situations in view of the very rapid ball and player interchanges, and also the need for many fast limb and whole body actions. Ice hockey and handball are also very good – but not so popular.

TABLE TENNIS

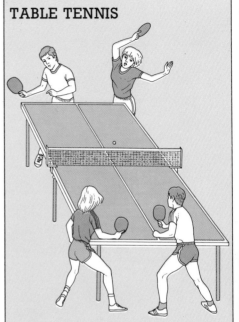

Table tennis is an excellent game for stimulus – response training and high speed movement. It is also an easy game to set up at home, requiring much less space than most physical games and inexpensive equipment. For more speed and fun try playing doubles. If possible, have a fifth person present to act as a referee, to control the scoring and spot errors.

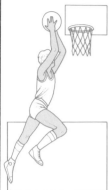

Basketball▲
One of the fastest of indoor games, basketball is used as a training exercise by athletes from many different sports. As a conclusion to a circuit training session it is ideal.

Karate▶
Although based on one of the most dangerous of martial arts, karate in sport is judged on skill, technique, timing and attitude – not on a competitor's ability to fell his opponent. Only the lightest of contact is permitted.

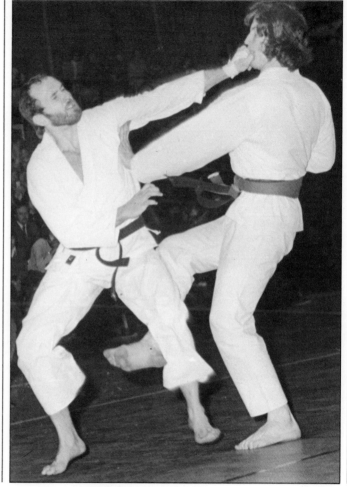

61

Stamina programmes

The components
You will recall that on pages 32–33, we saw that three major components of stamina training were Muscles, Circulation and Mind.

The muscle
The muscle stores fuel. During training it also improves its ability to transfer fuel from, and waste products to, the blood vessels which serve it.

Circulation
The heart as a pump becomes bigger, stronger, and more efficient – and increases its own network of blood vessels as well. The lungs become more effective due to the greater flexibility of the chest, and the strengthening of the muscles of breathing.

Mind
The philosopher said 'I think, therefore I am'. The trainer takes that one stage further 'I think I can, therefore I do'.
In a training programme which is progressive and successful, the mind is constantly reaching forward to the next objective, assessing and evaluating it, and preparing the body for what it knows can be achieved.

MUSCLE

As we have seen, there are two types of muscle fibre: fast and slow. The fast fibres are bigger than the slow ones but they use less oxygen and have a smaller blood supply. Slow muscle fibres, although less strong, have a much larger blood supply and much greater capacity for storing energy and consuming oxygen. They release their energy very slowly over long periods.

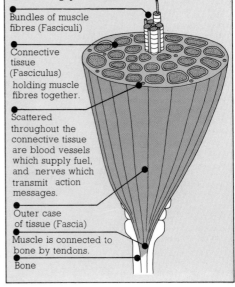

Bundles of muscle fibres (Fasciculi)

Connective tissue (Fasciculus) holding muscle fibres together.

Scattered throughout the connective tissue are blood vessels which supply fuel, and nerves which transmit action messages.

Outer case of tissue (Fascia)

Muscle is connected to bone by tendons.

Bone

CIRCULATION

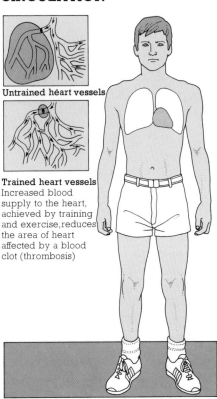

Untrained heart vessels

Trained heart vessels
Increased blood supply to the heart, achieved by training and exercise, reduces the area of heart affected by a blood clot (thrombosis)

Through stamina training, the capillaries of the heart interconnect to increase the blood routes through the heart.

MIND

The greatest advances in human performance are coming now because of psychological training. The key to unlock the great strong room of each individual's potential lies in his mind.

Increased physical performance confronts the individual with barriers, by training it is possible to shift the psychological barrier a great deal further towards the physiological barrier – in fact until they are at the same point. Some extremely highly motivated people can work until they lose consciousness, and in the superfit healthy person no harm is caused by doing so. Most people's psychological barrier is at a ludicrously low level. Stamina training can, and should, shift it a long way without getting anywhere near blackout levels.

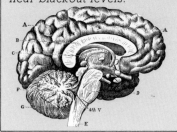

Stamina clothing

Stamina training involves the burning of a great deal of energy. This creates heat, and one becomes very warm. To allow this heat to dissipate, little clothing should be worn. If training outdoors, the clothing should be white or light coloured in order to reflect heat from the sun – and also to be more visible if training in traffic. Clothing should be loose and well ventilated to allow air to pass over the skin. String vests are very good for this, and cotton materials which allow sweat to permeate.

Footwear

This is specific to the activity, but most stamina training involves running for which correct footwear is absolutely critical. Shoes should have a hard long lasting sole, with a good tread to avoid slipping. There should be a sandwich layer of soft resilient material which will absorb the repeated shock of foot hitting the ground with the whole bodyweight on it. There should also be a built-in medium arch support and an inner porous sock which is removable for washing and/or replacement when worn.

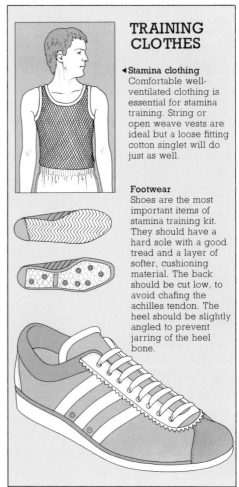

TRAINING CLOTHES

◀ **Stamina clothing**
Comfortable well-ventilated clothing is essential for stamina training. String or open weave vests are ideal but a loose fitting cotton singlet will do just as well.

Footwear
Shoes are the most important items of stamina training kit. They should have a hard sole with a good tread and a layer of softer, cushioning material. The back should be cut low, to avoid chafing the achilles tendon. The heel should be slightly angled to prevent jarring of the heel bone.

Stamina safety

Since stamina training varies from being the most to the least intense effort, the stresses it imposes are quite varied. The one which concerns most people is the stress on the heart.

The heart
In a healthy heart, free from defects, there is no possibility of overstrain through training. Particularly if the methods described in this book are followed, people with a clean bill of health medically can undertake stamina training without fear.

Individuals suffering from an infection which raises body temperature should not train for stamina. It is particularly common for athletes suffering from influenza to 'run it off', but the practice is not advised.

It is now fairly common practice even for heart patients to undertake carefully supervised stamina training in order to prevent another coronary from striking them. But, if you are overweight, over 40, or have parents who suffered heart disease, get a thorough medical before starting training.

The joints
Highly repetitive running routines can cause inflammation and arthritic changes in the ankle and knee joints particularly. This is most prevalent in those who run mainly on hard surfaces such as tarmacadam roads. Good shoes help to prevent this, but so also does running on soft surfaces, and developing a low shuffling running style like marathon runners.

The skin
Blisters are a constant problem, whether on the feet of the runner, or the bottom of the cyclist. Daily rubbing with spirits can help, but natural hardening is the best in the long term. When blisters arrive on the feet, pierce with a sterilised needle, express all the fluid, and tape firmly with one layer of thin non-stretch adhesive tape. Leave for a week or more before removal of the tape. For cyclist's bottom, use 'plastic skin' rather than tape.

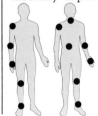

Ailments
Most healthy people will not experience heart trouble during stamina training, but blisters, soreness and joint inflammation are common problems.

The attitude to stamina

Training is based on overload. Overload involves making tasks more difficult. In this 'labour saving' age, we are hellbent on making tasks easier. It seems faintly ridiculous to be presented with opportunity for stamina training in one situation, only to reject it and use up valuable time elsewhere for stamina training. For example, anyone working on a high floor in a building has at least 2 opportunities per day to do some interval training by sprinting up 1 or 2 flights of stairs, resting, doing 2 more, resting, and so on. That consumes very little extra time, if any.

The journey to work represents another golden opportunity to do stamina training by fast walking, running, cycling or even roller skating! Frequently travelling time can be cut, and there are great financial savings.

It just requires that you build up a positive attitude to your own stamina development.

DIET FOR THE BIG EVENT

Occasionally we face a stiff test of stamina which cannot be described as training – something at which we want to perform to our best. It might be a sponsored marathon of some description, or a challenge walk over mountains, or a long distance race. Scientists have devised a special diet which can double the fuel stores in the muscles. This delays significantly the onset of fatigue, and reduces the amount of food you need to take during the test. In essence, it involves first starving yourself of carbohydrate, then gorging yourself on it. The muscles become so anxious to get fuel that they greedily stuff much more than usual into their storage spaces. No harm is suffered using this diet, though diabetics ought not to use it.

SUNDAY/MONDAY/TUESDAY	WEDNESDAY/THURSDAY/FRIDAY	SATURDAY
MEAT, FISH, EGGS, DAIRY PRODUCE **Train to exhaustion on a high protein diet**	CEREALS, PEAS/BEANS, SUGAR POTATOES, PUDDINGS, PASTRY **Reduce protein and cram the muscles with carbohydrate**	★LIGHT MEAL **Performance Day**

★ Eat a light meal at least two hours before event

Muscle stamina

The essence of muscle stamina training has the time honoured title of 'getting the miles in'. In short, thousands and thousands of repetitions of the movement. It is mistakenly thought that sportsmen exhibit the greatest stamina, but that is just not true. For example, the shop assistant who stands with little movement all day has stamina of the back postural muscles which no athlete could match. And what about a typist, who would think nothing of making up to 100,000 finger movements in a full day? Far more individual muscle actions than any marathon cyclist or runner. Whatever the training target, it is expressed in terms of 'how long' and 'how hard' – and the methods of training are the same. The early stages of training involve increasing gradually the rate at which you are working until you are able to comfortably to work at the target rate. This might be running at 7mph, or cycling at 15mph, or hill walking at 2mph, or typing at 40 words per minute, or whatever.

The early training also includes increasing gradually the length of time you can keep going non-stop until you are able fairly comfortably to work for the target time. This might be anything from 5 minutes to 10 hours. Then these two are combined by gradually extending the 'work rate' sessions in length, and intensifying the work rate in the 'length' sessions. Eventually the progress in each will coincide, and you will have achieved your target. You may stick at that – or set a new even higher target. There are no theoretical limits to how fit you can become!

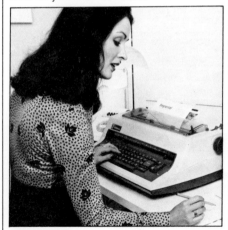

Muscle stamina
Any muscle which is required to make many repetitions of the same action must have stamina. A typist may make 100,000 finger movements in one day.

Circuit training

This is a very popular form of training. The theory is quite simple. Since the heart has more endurance than any other muscle in the body, any exercise tires out the movement muscle before tiring the heart. If you are doing consecutive sets of one particular exercise, when you stop to let your muscles recover, your heart rate is nowhere near its peak, and recovers almost to its starting point again. The first graph on page 71 shows this effect.

In circuit training, however, when you finish a set of one exercise you transfer immediately to another exercise which uses different (fresher) muscles, and keep working just as hard. By the time you have changed again to a third or fourth muscle group, the original group will have recovered and be ready to go again. The second graph shows that the heart remains exercised all the time, and eventually the heart rate reaches really high levels – indicating that the heart is working hard. It does not need to remain at this level very long. Even ten minutes are enough.

A bonus of circuit training is that strength and power exercises can be used, thus developing strength, speed and stamina simultaneously. A typical circuit of bodyweight exercises is shown in the chart opposite.

Once through this circuit would take anything from 3 minutes upwards, and would be sufficient for a beginner. The beauty of the system is that any exercise can be used, with any equipment and in any place.

Most people find that they make rapid progress, so that they are able to go round the circuit 2 or 3 times without stopping. Also, since they are becoming stronger they can do more repetitions of each exercise, maybe spending longer on each one. This means that the total time spent on a session by a really fit person might be as much as 20 minutes, with the heart rate perhaps well over 180 beats per minute.

Group circuits

With good organisation it is possible for there to be as many people working on a given circuit as the number of exercises in it. One person calls 'Change' every 30 or 60 seconds, and everyone changes to the next exercise simultaneously. There must be no hold ups on the change, the same equipment (if any) being used by all. This is a 'time dependent' circuit, and each person works flat out at each exercise for the whole time rather than a certain number of repetitions. It is also helpful if the exercises are laid out in a circle, so that people can move round (in the same direction) without confusion. Multistation machines are ideal for this form of group training, taking up to 12 people simultaneously.

Competition

Competition makes circuit training more enjoyable and beneficial. Solo circuit training is the best form of competition: a number of repetitions at each exercise are specified and each individual is timed for total circuit(s). If different targets are set for each exercise (e.g. beginner, moderate and super), individuals can be promoted from the lower to the higher circuits as their times improve.

WORKING A CIRCUIT

Circuit training
A circuit of exercises can be improvised in any reasonable amount of space, but without gymnasium equipment most of the exercises would have to be bodyweight or suppleness exercises.

EXERCISE	NUMBER OF REPETITIONS	SPECIFIC EXERCISE
Shuttle run	160 metres (175 yards)	*Legs*
Press-ups	20 repetitions	*Arm extension*
Sit ups	30 repetitions	*Trunk flexion*
High jumps	30 repetitions	*Leg extension*
Chin the bar	15 repetitions	*Arm flexion*
Back raises	30 repetitions	*Trunk extension*
Squat thrusts	30 repetitions	*Whole body*

●**Shuttle run**
A sprint over several lengths of the gymnasium, or circuit area, involving fast turns at each end.

●**Press ups and sit ups**
Standard exercises in any circuit; find them on pages 42 and 43.
Back raises
See 'Trunk extend' page 43.

●**High jumps**
From squatting position, or from a standing position bringing knees up to the chest.
●**Chin the bar**
See page 42.

●**Squat thrusts**
Keeping your hands on the floor, jump forwards to bring your knees level with your elbows. 'Thrust' your feet back to the starting position and repeat.

Interval training

Whereas the aim of circuit training is to develop the performance of the heart during sustained work, *interval training's* effect on the heart is to improve its ability to recover from hard work. As its name suggests, there are rest intervals built into the training, which is generally some form of locomotion like running or swimming, long enough to allow the first fairly steep heart recovery to take place. The rest interval should not be too long, otherwise the gradually increasing demand on the heart (and its recovery) will not be maintained.

In a well structured interval training session, the heart rate should behave as illustrated in the graph. Of course, the precise length of work sessions and the corresponding rest intervals may vary a great deal. They depend on the nature of the work to be performed (long or short bursts, high or lower level activity) and the type of rest period which would normally be expected.

For example, a boxer's interval training should provide him with 2–3 minute sessions of very hard work, with rest intervals of 30–45 seconds. On the other hand, a soccer player's sessions should be much shorter, since he rarely works hard continuously for more than a minute (and usually for much less), but may have to recover within ten or twenty seconds.

There is no reason why interval training sessions should not last for an hour or more. On the other hand sprint and middle distance performers frequently use interval training, working short distances at their desired racing pace in order to benefit their speed, and reducing the rest intervals until they disappear. They can then maintain the target pace for the whole distance.

Faartlek
This is a Scandinavian word meaning 'speed play'. It represents a less formal kind of interval training devised originally by those who ran in the beautiful forests and hills of that region. A fairly lengthy run is performed, of an hour or more, varying the pace a great deal, but including a reasonable proportion of fast running. Frequent stops are made, either for recovery or to take some other form of exercise – including games or relay races. Though faartlek can be a very casual kind of training,

the actual make up of the session can be structured very precisely in order to achieve quite specific training aims.

Games

Nearly all physical games constitute a form of interval training. Play is intermittent with frequent rest pauses, and may vary greatly in intensity. Most games last for upwards of 30 minutes and some, like tennis are not time restricted – so that the players could be involved for 5 hours or more. When interval training is used as a means of training to play games it must be structured so as to resemble the game, but more intense. But when games are used as means to achieve good fitness, then they become the most enjoyable form of interval training.

In this case, the game must be played intensively – even to the stage where the exercise is more important than the result! After a particularly tough burst of activity, the temptation is to take an extended pause, and to cruise for a while until recovery is complete. This is tactically sensible when playing in a game where the result is the most important thing, but self defeating when playing for fitness.

TRAINING HEART RATES

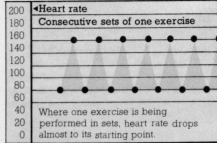

◄Heart rate
Consecutive sets of one exercise

Where one exercise is being performed in sets, heart rate drops almost to its starting point.

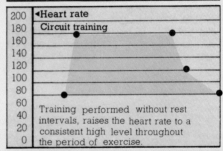

◄Heart rate
Circuit training

Training performed without rest intervals, raises the heart rate to a consistent high level throughout the period of exercise.

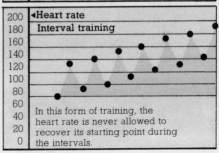

◄Heart rate
Interval training

In this form of training, the heart rate is never allowed to recover its starting point during the intervals.

Suppleness programmes

Anatomy

The joints and muscles with which we are concerned here are distributed throughout the body. The ones you work on in a stamina programme will depend upon what you want the suppleness for. A track athlete will want moderate all-round suppleness, a rower will be chiefly concerned with the shoulders and lower back, a gymnast will possess extreme suppleness of the spine, abdomen and hips. For general fitness, exceptional suppleness is not necessary – nor desirable.

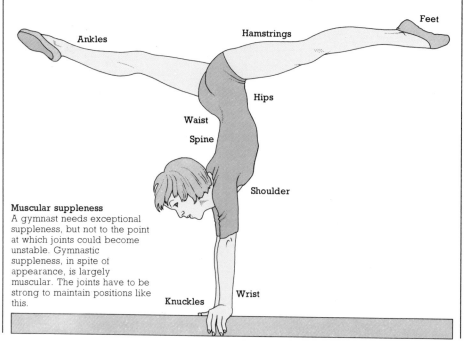

Muscular suppleness

A gymnast needs exceptional suppleness, but not to the point at which joints could become unstable. Gymnastic suppleness, in spite of appearance, is largely muscular. The joints have to be strong to maintain positions like this.

Suppleness safety

Suppleness training is potentially harmful, and every item of training needs to be undertaken with great care. Too much suppleness is worse than too little. The latter will merely hamper performance and occasionally lead to pulled muscles. The former leads to joint instability and the danger of arthritic changes in the joint.

Additionally, the development of suppleness depends on stretching muscles and ligaments, which is in itself a dangerous process. Because of this, all suppleness training should be preceded by a warm up, and the warmth maintained by wearing warm clothes. These should not constrain the movements being performed.

The guidelines of safety are set by pain. Stretching exercises must of necessity be uncomfortable, but they should never produce sharp pain. Progressive forces must be applied from each movement to the next, leading to gradually increasing stretch on each movement. The rate of increase will be greater when stretching muscle than with ligament. Do not overstretch muscles or ligaments which have been recently injured.

DISPERSING TENDERNESS

Suppleness sessions frequently lead to great tenderness in the muscles concerned. This can be dispersed more quickly by applying deep heat, gentle stretching, skilful massage, warm baths or elevating the limbs. Though not harmful in itself, the discomfort produced by the tenderness can cause normal body movements to be changed in such a way as to make injury more likely.

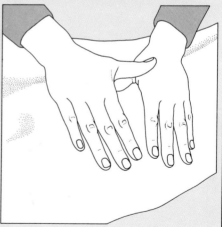

Massage
Tenderness can be dispersed by massage provided that the practitioner is sufficiently skilled.

Joint exercises

The following pages contain a number of exercises for improving the suppleness of neck, shoulder, spine, hips, ankle and wrist. All of these exercises should be performed smoothly and steadily, with no sudden movements. Never force a joint, especially if you can feel pain. Joint exercises are best undertaken in conjunction with other suppling exercises

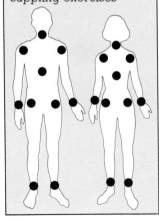

NECK

Though neck mobility is limited by bony structures in the forward and backwards directions, it is beneficial to increase the sideways and rotational mobility by gentle stretching.

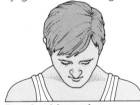

Drop head forward

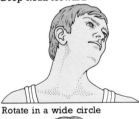

Rotate in a wide circle

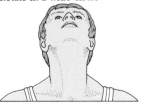

Repeat in the other direction

SHOULDER

The shoulder is a very complicated joint, and we tend to concentrate on the movements themselves. The two important ones are rotation, and extension behind the head.

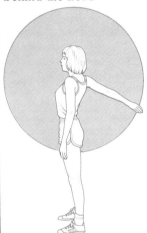

Trace large circles with the arms

As an alternative to the exercise shown, try extending both arms simultaneously backwards and upwards to reach head level.

SPINE

The important suppleness here is in the backward extension of the lower spine, the forward and sideways flexion and the rotation of the whole spine.

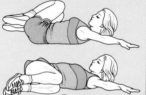

Rotation▲
Keep the body flat on the floor and move only from the hips. This one is best performed on a mat.

Forward flexion▼
There are many variations on this, in both standing and sitting positions.

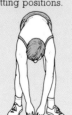

Sideways flexion▼
Can also be a rotational exercise, when it includes extension.

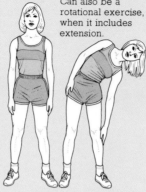

Backward extension▼
This can also be done in a kneeling or sitting position.

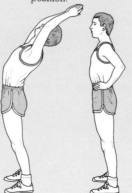

HIP

The hip is a very strong joint, with a small possibility of increasing sideways mobility. But, leg split mobility can be extensive, and with great care various exercises can achieve surprisingly good results.

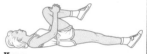

Knee press

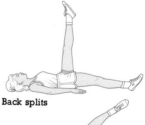

Back splits

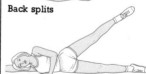

Side splits

The best hip exercises are all variations on leg splits.

HAND

The knuckle joints benefit by flexibility in all directions, but finger joints should not normally be tampered with.

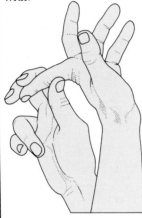

Elbow Knee

There can be no good reason for increasing normal mobility. There are certain joints which should not, except when undergoing physiotherapy, be subjected to suppleness exercises.

WRIST

Both forward flexion and backward extension should be developed at least to a 90° angle.

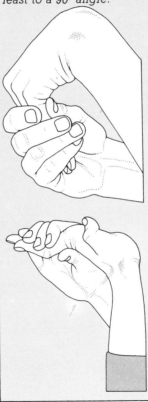

ANKLE/FOOT

The ankle should have a reasonable amount of mobility in all directions, though much of this mobility comes from the foot joints rather than the ankle.

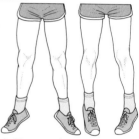

Ankle extension
With your feet 6in(15cm) apart, rise on your toes lifting your heels as high as you can. Do it first with toes pointing in and then pointing out. Repeat 30 times.

Foot

Like the hand, it is beneficial to increase the mobility of the knuckle joints, but also some of the toes may well repay some exercise.

Whole movements

In actual physical performance we usually make whole movements which involve more than one joint, and the muscles which act across joints. The exercises so far have been designed to isolate joints so that the effects are quite specific. But when doing whole movements it is possible to compensate for immobility in one area by greater mobility in another. Shown here are a range of exercises for whole movements: Forward Bending, Backward Bending, Twisting, and Splits. These basic exercises, with many variations to suit each individual, form a bedrock of general suppleness training. They should be done daily if possible, just using an odd few minutes here and there.

Split movements
This movement, often called the hurdlers exercise, develops flexibility of the hips, spine and hamstrings.

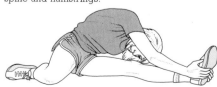

ALL-ROUND EXERCISES

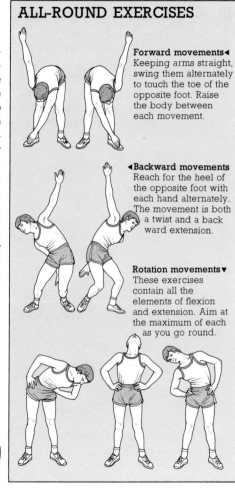

Forward movements◄
Keeping arms straight, swing them alternately to touch the toe of the opposite foot. Raise the body between each movement.

◄Backward movements
Reach for the heel of the opposite foot with each hand alternately. The movement is both a twist and a backward extension.

Rotation movements▼
These exercises contain all the elements of flexion and extension. Aim at the maximum of each as you go round.

Partner work

Some people who are very stiff do not have the skill or sensitivity in their joints and muscles which allows them to stretch themselves fully. They are inhibited from extreme positions. This is particularly true in people whose stiffness is due to injury. Working carefully with a partner (helper) can overcome this problem. Partners must remember that movements should always be gradual. One person cannot feel the pain experienced by the other, and it is easy to stretch one's partner too far.

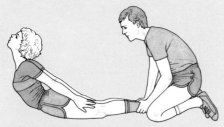

Working with your partner
This is a very difficult exercise to perform well without a partner. As in all partner work, the job of the assistant is to help the other person carry out the exercise properly, not to make it more difficult.

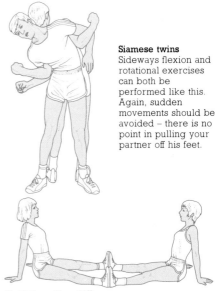

Siamese twins
Sideways flexion and rotational exercises can both be performed like this. Again, sudden movements should be avoided – there is no point in pulling your partner off his feet.

Splitting the difference
The object is to push against the other person's feet, gradually widening the leg-split.

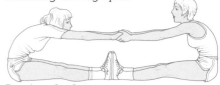

Rowing the boat
Rock backwards and forwards with regular, even resistance. Do not make sudden jerky movements.

Suppleness in ordinary living

We are born very supple, and retain this through early childhood while we still perform movements which explore the limits of our physical potential. Then, gradually, our lifestyle becomes physically more conservative. We avoid extreme body positions and our suppleness is eroded. Yet it need not be. Some quite ancient people still retain phenomenal flexibility. There is no natural law which says 'Old is Stiff'. Within our daily activities we have the opportunity to stretch ourselves. Shown are some ways of doing it:

Bend down

Although heavy weights ought not to be lifted with the legs straight and the back bent, work at floor level can be performed in this position. In the early days keep the feet wide apart, bringing them closer as suppleness increases.

Bend back

Man is a frontal animal, and does most actions in front of the body. He could profit by taking a leaf from the book of other animals – Stretch up and back, at least to retrieve objects if placing them is too difficult.

Twist yourself

The swivel chair should be jettisoned. Make your spine and shoulders do some stretching for a change. The same applies when ironing, or even washing your own back.

EVERYDAY EXERCISES

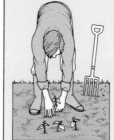

◄**Forward flexion**
Gardening is one of those everyday tasks which could be useful exercise. When working at ground level, keep the legs straight and bend from the waist.

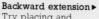

Backward extension▶
Try placing and retrieving objects by bending backwards to reach them. It may not always be practical, but it can make chores more fun to do. After all, fitness and fun do go together.

Skill programmes

We have already seen that most fitness elements contribute to the overall skill of human performance. Particularly, that speed fitness includes the development of skill in detecting and processing information. So, at this stage we will concern ourselves with skill defined as 'the similarity between intention and achievement'. Somewhere in our mind's eye there is a 'picture' of the movement we intend to perform. The difference between that and the actual movement we perform represents a lack of skill.

We must not be confused by a movement which achieves the desired effect – like scoring a goal, or threading a needle – but more by luck than skill, or despite a lack of skill. The way in which the result is obtained is also important. Equally we must beware of developing highly skilful actions which do not achieve the desired end result.

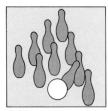

Achievement
The bowler's skill does not match his perception of the game.

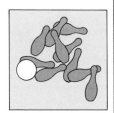

Intention
The gap between this and the achievement represents a lack of skill.

Objective skill▶
The intention of a ten-pin bowler is quite clear: to knock down the maximum number of pins in one delivery. He may see this vividly in his mind's eye, but he will not have mastered the skill until he can perform the action without referring to his mental picture.

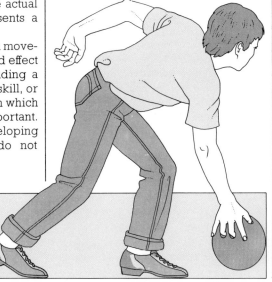

Skill training

For some reason, skill training is called *practice*, and the most important saying is 'Practice makes perfect'. But practice only perfects the exact movement which is being practised. If that movement is imperfect (unskilful), then 'Practice makes *imperfect*'. And, trying to correct bad faults later on is a very difficult business.

Knowledge of results

When acquiring skill the human acts as a control system. If the result of each practice movement is not known, then the following movement cannot be modified. Even if the results are known after every few practices, it is difficult to achieve precise modification. The ideal is to know the result immediately after every action. This may be easy to check for yourself, or you may need someone to help you. When the result *is* the movement, it is not really possible to see yourself properly, so you need a skilled observer to help you, and/or a video tape recorder, to give instant feedback.

This knowledge should adapt our performance. The effect will be re-inforced if reward and penalty are used carefully. A good movement would be praised and a bad one penalised (by scorn or penalty). For example, if a hundred repetitions are being done a target of sixty successful ones might be set. Each repetition could receive verbal praise or criticism, and the whole session be rewarded or penalised depending on the achievement of the target.

Monitoring performance
A video recording is the best means of analysing your own performance. The feedback is instant and accurate. Failing that, a skilled and knowledgeable observer will serve you well.

Speed versus accuracy

Speed is not important in all movements. For example, the speed at which the dart is thrown into the dartboard is similar for most players, and they do not attempt to increase that speed. There is no trade-off between speed and accuracy. The opposite is the case in tennis serving, where the faster you serve the less accurately can you place and spin the ball.

Where there is trade-off, practice must always be as accurate as possible building up the speed gradually.

Spacing

'Little and often' is the best rule for acquiring new skill. If you are going to do 1,000 repetitions of a movement in a week (and that is not very many!) then 5 days of 4 sessions of 5 sets of 10 repetitions is far better than 2 days of 2 sessions of 2 sets of 250 repetitions. Especially when developing new skills, *do not practice when tired* since that changes the skill and leads to bad habits.

Trying too hard

There is a famous law discovered by Yerkes-Dodson which describes the effects on skill of trying too hard, particularly through overmotivation. The message is, try to find the right amount of motivation. Too much is as bad as too little!

Closed versus open

Be careful to distinguish between those skills which are almost identical each time you do them – like dart throwing, or plain stitch in knitting – to those which are unique solutions to unique situations – like a goal scored in soccer. The closed skills are practised in a highly repetitive 'grooved' fashion, doing away with the brain altogether; whereas the open skills are developed in an adaptable way, with full mental participation and in sight. Most skills have a bit of both in them, so the early training is done in a closed fashion, moving to open principles as the skill becomes 'grooved'.

Assisted training ▶
The parade ground method of 'follow me' instruction is not very satisfactory from the individual point of view. But in small specialised groups, the presence of a coach or demonstrator can be of great benefit.

Assisted training

It is a very well known phenomenon that even quite ordinary people can experience brief moments of superb skill after watching champions in action. It is almost as if seeing the 'ultimate' releases the little bit of magic which lies within us all. Certainly the 'Follow me' method of teaching skills has been favoured for many years, where a good performer will do the movement, being shadowed by the learner. It is, of course, vital that the demonstration should be as perfect as possible. One danger of shadow practice is that the technique of the demonstrator is specific to him, to his levers and reactions and personality. The learner may not be suited to that identical movement, so quite soon after learning by shadow practice the learner should practice on his own in order to develop his own style.

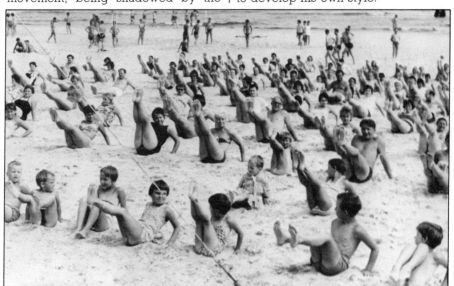

Kinaesthesis

This word has not been inserted just to frighten the reader. There is no other word which will do to explain 'the sense of where you are', which is of vital importance in skill training. Though shadow practice can give the learner a mental image of the desired movement, and some idea of its timing it gives him no idea of what the movement feels like.

The mental computer has a great deal of information from outside the body which defines where it is 'in space'. Mainly from the eyes, you know which way you face and whether you

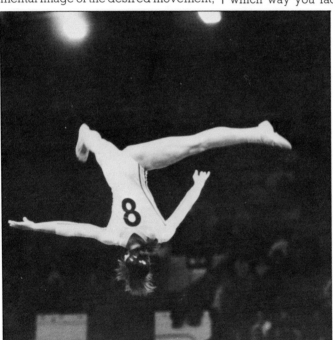

Kinaesthesis
The gymnast or acrobat demonstrates the perfect working of kinaesthesis. In this picture, the gymnast, although upside down, retains a precise understanding of where she is in relation to her surroundings. She knows how and where she will come down and is capable of repeating the exercise many times. Partly by training the eyes to certain fixed points, and partly by knowing what every position feels like, she manages to remain in control throughout the movement.

are upside down. But even with the eyes closed, you can tell if you are upside down because of special sense organs in the head.

The head in fact, provides a reference point from which the computer can tell the position of every other body part. All joints and muscles have special sensors in them which build up this total picture in the brain. For skills which involve knowing where you are in space, like doing somersaults or fast spins, the eyes should be fixed on some point and return to it as soon as possible after having moved.

When learning new movements, it can help if a teacher manipulates the learner's body through the action, so that the computer can begin to build up the correct model of what the movement feels like. But, like shadow practice, the learner needs to be left on his own quite soon so that his style becomes a personal one.

It also helps to practice some movements without looking at them, as soon as possible after they have been learned. Eventually you should not need to use the eyes to *perform* any movement skilfully, but only to relate that movement to your surroundings.

PRESSURE TRAINING

One of the frustrating aspects of skill training is what happens when a skill which has been well learned in training is suddenly exposed to the pressure of competition, or critical scrutiny, or fatigue. The skill breaks down.

Quite obviously, skill training is not complete without sessions which apply pressure on the performer. And yet this is often neglected. Ball games offer the best opportunities for pressure training because it is easier to simulate and intensify the pressures of competition than it is in, say, shot putting or high diving. A good example of how pressure can be applied is the game known as the 'pepperpot'. In this, several players form a circle around the one who is to be pressured. A ball is passed to the player in the centre who passes to the next in the circle who passes back to the centre. The centre player is the only one to move the ball on. Pressure is applied by feeding a second ball in just after the first, so that the centre player is always receiving and returning the first ball and about to receive the second.

Body shape

The Narcissus complex

Many of us who become extremely fit are not satisfied with knowing it ourselves. We want other people to know it as well, and yet it gets a bit boring if you have to *tell* everyone how fit you are. Much better, in fact, to be an obvious example of good fitness – not only for the ego, but also as an advertisement for fitness itself.

It is not surprising that a commonly used phrase to describe fitness is 'being in shape'. Though you cannot see the heart and lungs, the body cannot lie about its fitness. You look what you are. And in all walks of life, a person who looks a picture of health and fitness inspires confidence which is to his credit in the overall assessment made of him.

As sculptors, given the lump of clay which is our bodies, how can we create a masterpiece? Well, there are two materials (fat and muscle), and the way they hang together (posture).

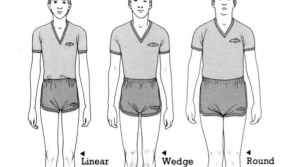

Linear   Wedge   Round

Basic body shapes
Whether we like it or not, our bodies are simply developments of the natural shapes that we were born with. The three basic patterns of human shape, linear, wedge and round, are shown here.

1. Linear (sometimes called **Ectomorph**) Angular, lean, probably having plenty of stamina but not much muscle.

2. Wedge (Mesomorph)
Muscular, wide shouldered, energetic, but needs exercise to keep in shape.

3. Round (Endomorph)
Large boned and well rounded, tendency to put on weight easily, exercise very necessary.

FAT SPOTS

The critical spots from which fat must be trimmed are easily identified. Though diet will reduce fat generally, it can't get at the specific sites. So you need to supplement your diet by exercising the muscles in and on which the unwanted fat is deposited. Massage and localised sweating does not get rid of local fat deposits.

Muscle

This is body building for the sake of appearance. What one person thinks is an attractive body, may be unpleasant to another. So the body you build should fit your own view of what is desirable.

If we examine the body, we can see those parts where good muscle development and size are desirable; and where the overall shape of the body can most easily be changed.

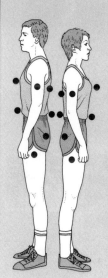

Critical fat spots
The following locations are the places in which fat is most likely to build up – and develop an unsatisfactory body shape. Nearly everybody can reduce weight with a combination of diet and exercise.

1. Breast/chest	●
2. Stomach	●
3. Waist	●
4. Back	●
5. Buttocks	●
6. Thighs	●
7. Upper Arms	●

Muscle zones
The areas indicated are those which most readily show the benefits of exercise. It is up to each individual to decide how much muscle development is desirable.

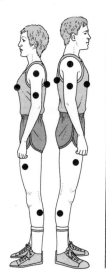

1. Shoulder	●
2. Back	●
3. Upper Arms	●
4. Breast	●
5. Chest	●
6. Thighs	●
7. Calf	●

Posture

In some ways, posture is a matter of fashion. The Army has one fashion, discomaniacs have another, fashion models differ from both. These are specialist postures, each of which has some undesirable elements in it.

Perhaps the best criterion of general posture should be health and function. Our bodies should spend most of their time in postures which do not cause 'self inflicted' wear and tear, and which permit us to function efficiently.

The postures shown can be developed by strengthening the muscles which support the various joints concerned, and by developing the mental attitude which ensures that the posture is continuously consciously corrected – until it becomes second nature.

GOOD POSTURE

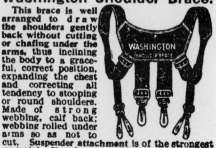

Everyday good posture
Make a conscious effort to keep your spine straight and head upright. Distribute your weight evenly on both feet, stand erect and confidently but not stiffly to attention.

BAD HABITS

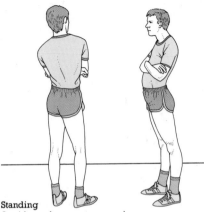

Standing
Avoid careless posture, such as the common habit of resting one leg and stooping, and slackening the spine. These postures can affect the muscles controlling body alignment.

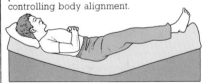

Resting
Sagging and soft mattresses and poorly sprung bed frames can affect posture and cause back trouble. There is no need to sleep on boards but choose firm, supportive mattresses. Remember to sit correctly, avoiding the habits of lounging and stooping forwards.

Weekly schedules

Overleaf are some suggested training schedules for four representative people of different age groups, male or female. Many people will want to make up their own, more specific, schedules; we can only suggest general fitness programmes with varying degrees of emphasis. They will, however, give you some idea of how a schedule can be made up and how to adapt one for your own use.

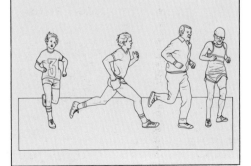

AGES 12-19

You may be committed to a certain number of activities as part of your regular fitness programme. In addition, cycling, running, or some kind of competitive ball game can be substituted in the appropriate places for the games and sports in the programme.

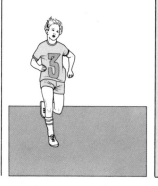

WEEKLY SCHEDULE

	Morning	Afternoon	Evening
Monday	Cycle to school 4 miles	Lunch-time circuit training	Cycle home 4 miles
Tuesday	Cycle to school 4 miles	Midday suppleness and strength session	Cycle home Badminton club evening
Wednesday	Cycle to school 4 miles	Football or hockey training afternoon	Cycle home
Thursday	Cycle to school 4 miles		Cycle home Badminton club evening
Friday	Cycle to school 4 miles	Suppleness and strength session midday	Cycle home
Saturday	Football or Hockey competitive match		Disco evening
Sunday		90 minute cycle ride fairly hard	

AGES 20-40

This programme is based on one session each day, the time restrictions of people in this age group being the most severe. The level of activity will depend upon the commitment of the individual, but it is reasonable to assume that one hour each day is the maximum of time available.

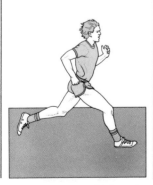

WEEKLY SCHEDULE

	Morning	Afternoon	Evening
Monday		Lunchtime speed and interval training session	
Tuesday			Club training including circuit and skill session
Wednesday	Suppleness training session		
Thursday			Club training including circuit and skill session
Friday	Suppleness training session		
Saturday		Basketball or rugby competitive match	
Sunday	Two hour run		

AGES 40-65

In this age group, regularity of fitness activities and structuring of programmes becomes important if fitness is not to go by the board. Although suppleness and stamina may appear to be more important than they were at an earlier age, speed should not be neglected – especially if you have always been involved in speed activities.

WEEKLY SCHEDULE

	Morning	Afternoon	Evening
Monday	Walk or cycle to work		Suppleness and strength session
Tuesday	Walk or cycle to work	Suppleness session Squash match	
Wednesday	Walk or cycle to work		Suppleness session or Keep fit class
Thursday	Walk or cycle to work	Suppleness session Squash match	
Friday	Walk or cycle to work		Suppleness and strength session
Saturday		Heavy gardening or decorating	
Sunday	Suppleness session	Run/walk faartlek 75 minutes	

AGES 65 plus

There is no reason why, at pensionable age, you should not be able to do the things you could do when you were younger. You will, inevitably, be slower but there is no reason why your strength and suppleness should be overlooked. At this age, playing golf and taking long walks may be more valuable than they were when you were younger.

WEEKLY SCHEDULE

	Morning	Afternoon	Evening
Monday	Suppleness and strength session	One hour swimming	
Tuesday	Suppleness and strength session	9–18 holes golf	
Wednesday	Suppleness and strength session		One hour swimming
Thursday	Suppleness and strength session	9–18 holes golf	
Friday	Suppleness and strength session	One hour swimming	
Saturday	Gardening and/or social walk		
Sunday	Suppleness and strength session	Gardening session	

Index

●Figures in italics refer to illustrations

TERMINOLOGY

Antagonist
The muscles which oppose those performing an action are called the antagonist muscles.

Circuit training
A series of differing exercises, performed in sequence, without rest intervals.

Concentric
A muscular movement which overcomes resistance.

Eccentric
The movement caused when a muscle is overcome by resistance is called eccentric.

Interval training
Repeated sets of one exercise with rest intervals between. The object is to increase the heart rate gradually over the whole period of exercise until it reaches fairly high levels.

Kinaesthesis
The name given to the process performed by the human brain during complicated or acrobatic exercise which enables the athlete to retain an understanding of his relationship to his surroundings.

Stimulus-response
The speed of reaction of the brain to information received in the form of stimulus is an important aspect of many games and sports. It is known as the stimulus-response (S-R) mechanism.

Acknowledgments

The 'How To' Book of
Fitness and Exercise was
created by Simon Jennings
and Company Limited.
We are grateful to the
following individuals
and organisations for
their assistance in the
making of this book:

Mary Corcoran: *picture research*
John Couzins: *cover and title page photographs*
The Dover Archive: *engravings and embellishments*
Just Leisure Ltd, High Street, London S.E. 20, *sports equipment*
Coral Mula: *for all line and tone illustrations*
Anna Pavord: *compilation of index*
Helena Zakrsewska-Rucinska: *hand tinting of engravings*

Photographs:
Imperial Typewriters page **67**
Leo Mason pages **11** *tl*; **11** *b*; **23** *b*; **27** *b*; **31** *t*; **84**
Popperfoto page **83**
Spectrum Picture Library pages **6** *bl*; **22** *r*; **23** *tl*; **23** *tr*; **30** *bl*
Sport and General (Press Agency) Ltd. pages **37**; **40**; **56**; **61**
Daily Telegraph page **27** *t*
Zefa Picture Library pages **6** *bl*; **7** *t*; **7** *b*; **10** *tl*; **10** *bl*;
11 *tr*; **14** *bl*; **26** *tl*; **26** *bl*; **30** *tr*; **30** *br*; **31** *b*; **52/3**

abbreviations: *t* top; *b* bottom; *c* centre; *tl* top left; *tr* top right;
bl bottom left; *br* bottom right; *r* right

Typesetting by Servis Filmsetting Ltd., Manchester
Headline setting by Facet Photosetting, London

Special thanks to Norman Ruffell and
the staff of Swaingrove Ltd., Bury St. Edmunds,
Suffolk, for the lithographic reproduction.

'HOW TO'